THE POUND A DAY DIET

ALSO BY
ROCCO DISPIRITO

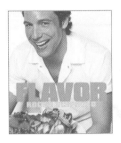

FLAVOR

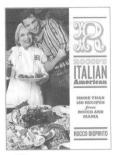

ROCCO'S ITALIAN-AMERICAN

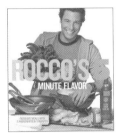

ROCCO'S FIVE MINUTE FLAVOR:
Fabulous Meals with 5 Ingredients in 5 Minutes

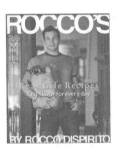

ROCCO'S REAL LIFE RECIPES:
Fast Flavor for Everyday

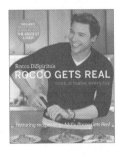

ROCCO GETS REAL:
Cook at Home Every Day

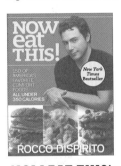

NOW EAT THIS!:
150 of America's Favorite Comfort Foods, All Under 350 Calories

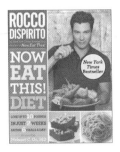

NOW EAT THIS! DIET:
Lose Up to 10 Pounds in Just 2 Weeks Eating 6 Meals a Day!

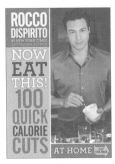

NOW EAT THIS! QUICK CALORIE CUTS:
At Home/On-the-Go

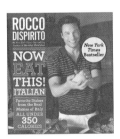

NOW EAT THIS! ITALIAN:
Favorite Dishes from the Real Mamas of Italy—All Under 350 Calories

THE POUND A DAY DIET

LOSE UP TO 5 POUNDS IN 5 DAYS BY EATING THE FOODS YOU LOVE

ROCCO DISPIRITO

GRAND CENTRAL
Life&Style
NEW YORK • BOSTON

GRAND CENTRAL LIFE & STYLE

Hachette Book Group
1290 Avenue of the Americas
New York, NY 10104
www.GrandCentralLifeandStyle.com

Printed in the United States of America

RRD-C

Originally published in hardcover by Hachette Book Group
First trade edition: February 2015

10 9 8 7 6 5 4 3 2 1

Grand Central Life & Style is an imprint of Grand Central Publishing.

The Grand Central Life & Style name and logo are trademarks of Hachette Book Group, Inc.

The Hachette Speakers Bureau provides a wide range of authors for speaking events. To find out more, go to www.hachettespeakersbureau.com or call (866) 376-6591.

The publisher is not responsible for websites (or their content) that are not owned by the publisher.

Design by Hsu + Associates

Library of Congress Cataloging-in-Publication Data

DiSpirito, Rocco.
    The pound a day diet : lose up to 5 pounds in 5 days by eating the foods you love / Rocco DiSpirito. — First edition.
        pages cm
    Includes index.
    ISBN 978-1-4555-2367-2 (hardback) — ISBN 978-1-4555-2369-6 (ebook)
    1. Reducing diets—Recipes. 2. Low-calorie diet—Recipes. 3. Self-care, Health. I. Title.
    RM222.2D5788 2014
    613.2′5—dc23
                                                                 2013030417

ISBN 978-1-4555-2368-9 (pbk.)

AUTHOR'S NOTE

This publication is intended to provide helpful and informative material on the subjects addressed. It is sold with the understanding that the author is not engaged in rendering medical, health, or any other kind of professional advice in the book. The reader should consult his or her own health care professional before adopting any of the suggestions in this book or drawing any inferences from it.

This book is not intended in any way to be a substitute for professional medical advice, diagnosis, or treatment. Never disregard professional medical advice or delay in seeking it because of something you have read in this book.

Notwithstanding the foregoing, the author has personally overseen and monitored participants in the Pound a Day Diet Plan exactly as specified in this book. Several of the participants provided testimonials included in this book. The results were astonishing. Over 95% of the participants who followed this program as specified lost 6 pounds of fat in the first week. Only one lost less than 5 pounds in the first week due to health related complications. All of the participants maintained or lost more weight after going off the diet. Results may not be typical.

DEDICATION

To The 300. You know who you are. You are true warriors whose weapons are your brilliant work and tireless pursuit of perfection. With every project we accomplish together you prove that fighting for your right to love what you do and do what you love is a battle that can be won every day.

And to the people in my test group for allowing me into their lives and for proving nothing is impossible.

Lose five pounds by friday!

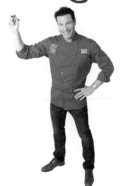

CONTENTS

RECIPE INDEX

MAIN COURSES

FOREWORD

THE BOOK you are holding in your hands represents a revolution in weight loss.

There has never been a diet book like *The Pound a Day Diet* before.

This is a totally new, breakthrough plan for losing weight.

It works because it is based on sound science and good nutrition, putting the principles of calorie control, calorie density, healthy rapid weight loss, whole foods, the Mediterranean diet pattern, and physical activity into an inspiring, delicious package that you can enjoy and that will get you to a healthy weight quickly and help you stay there over the long term.

In my medical practice, I have treated thousands of patients who were overweight or obese. I have seen the results of a host of failed diets: disappointing results and impossible-to-follow eating plans that are doomed to failure.

I have seen patients who have tried fad diets, crash diets, and gimmick diets based on bad science, and most of these patients have one thing in common: The diets fail, the weight bounces right back on and then some, and the patient becomes angry, depressed, and miserable. I don't blame them at all!

In talking to, counseling, and working with so many patients to help them achieve healthy weight over the long term, I have learned what works and what doesn't.

And *The Pound a Day Diet* works, for three striking reasons.

First, it was written by one of our country's great chefs, Rocco DiSpirito.

That means it is based on the kind of food you and your family not only can fall in love with, but will savor for the rest of your life. There are lots of diet books written by trainers and medical professionals, but only a master chef like Rocco can fully unlock for you the ultimate secret of a healthy, fast weight loss, which is flavor and satisfaction. Without that, I think most diets are doomed to fail.

I will now reveal to you one of the greatest diet secrets on earth. It is a revelation that I doubt any diet expert or doctor has ever told you. And Rocco has discovered this secret: **The ultimate diet is the one that gives you joy**.

The best diet for you is the healthy eating pattern that is based on the joy, pleasure, excitement, happiness, sexiness, energy, adventure, and peace that great food, lovingly prepared, gives you, so you can move to a healthy, lean food lifestyle for the rest of your life.

You should not suffer when you are on a diet. You should swoon. You should smile. You should enjoy yourself. And thanks to his knowledge, passion, and skill at creating inspiring cuisine, Rocco DiSpirito is a master of this experience. In this book, he will show you how easy it is for you to do this too, and how it can help you lose weight fast.

The second reason this diet will work for you is because it is based on the latest, cutting-edge science, which says that a dietary pattern based on whole, unprocessed foods in a calorie-corrected, healthy pattern like the Mediterranean diet is the key to both a long, healthy life and effective and lasting weight loss.

And third, **The Pound a Day Diet** is based on the major insight that fast, steady weight loss based on correctly balancing calorie intake, eating patterns, and physical activity, with a doctor's guidance, can for many people be highly motivating and inspiring. In my own practice, I have seen this formula prove to be effective and sustainable.

And on top of this, in this book, Rocco is pulling off no less than a diet miracle.

He is basing his diet on **real food**, on three square, nutritionally balanced meals a day, plus healthy snacks. And as someone who has savored Rocco's creations, I can tell you this food is spectacularly delicious.

Most diet books focus on foods you can't have. But **The Pound a Day Diet** focuses on what you can have and what you can savor.

That is the key to losing weight and keeping it off, and that's why this diet will work for you.

Jeffrey A. Morrison, MD, CNS

Founder of The Morrison Center for Integrative Medicine and award-winning
author of *Cleanse Your Body, Clear Your Mind*

INTRODUCTION

I USED to be a fat guy.

If you're struggling with your weight, I know exactly how you feel.

I was a chef who ate too much of his own merchandise.

I was sampling all the food I created. I spent most of my waking hours in a great restaurant surrounded by fantastic food, and I slowly packed on the pounds, lots of them. I started feeling self-conscious. And I was failing to take care of myself.

One day I looked down and could barely see my feet. My belly was partially blocking them.

I was only thirty-seven years old, but I was carrying an extra thirty pounds around on my body! My waist was crossing the thirty-eight-inch mark, and I was on a speeding freight train to emotional disaster, not to mention a host of likely medical problems like obesity, high blood pressure, diabetes, arthritis, and heart trouble, to name just a few.

What was my absolute worst moment?

It was the moment I realized I couldn't wear a regular chef's jacket anymore. I realized I had to get one with an extra-big belly sewn into it. Talk about humiliating! It was then that I knew I had to take control of the situation.

I immediately began a journey toward discovering the secrets of fast, effective, enjoyable weight loss. Crucially, I did this from a chef's perspective, from the perspective of someone who adores food and someone who savors every molecule of satisfaction food delivers. And that was one of the keys to my success. Savoring the healthy food I ate helped me lose the weight—and keep it off.

I melted the lard off my butt. I confronted it, crushed it, and defeated it. I clicked the Select All button on my body and reduced it by 15 percent. I deleted the extra tonnage, pressed the Empty Trash icon, and never looked back. Good-bye forever.

Today, the extra thirty pounds are gone, I've got a thirty-three- or thirty-four-inch waist, and I feel better than I ever felt before. I've felt this way for six years.

And the best part is, I don't deny myself delicious food and I don't torture myself over foods I "can't have" or foods I "have to give up." I love food, and man, do I eat it, all kinds of food, all times of day.

This book is about how you can do what I did, and do it quickly.

This is a revolutionary new diet approach that can help you lose as much as a pound of extra weight a day, and keep it off forever.

With my **Now Eat This!** series of books, I've helped hundreds of thousands of people cook their way to health with delicious, healthy recipes based on their favorite comfort foods. Those books have changed lives—so many that I've received tons of emails from readers. Many readers have asked for a program that delivers super-fast results—a program in which they do not necessarily need to cook and a plan that can fit into anyone's busy lifestyle. Readers wanted a program that they could start on Monday and be thinner for the weekend.

Well, I aim to please, so I began to research a new approach to weight loss based on the latest studies. **The Pound a Day Diet** is the result of that research. I discovered some amazing weight loss tips and secrets that I've used to create a fantastic, effective program.

You'll find the answer you've been searching for: lasting weight loss—without plateaus, without boredom, and without the urge to cheat. But that's only the beginning: Five days from now, you'll be looking in the mirror and seeing yourself trimmer, pounds lighter, and inches smaller.

This book can change your life.

It's a completely new approach to blasting off extra weight **and keeping it off for good**. **The Pound a Day Diet** is perfect for anyone who wants to:

- Be ready for an important weekend event or big date.
- Jump-start a weight loss program with fast and highly motivating results in five days.
- Fit into a wedding dress, prom gown, or tux.
- Drop those stubborn final pounds.
- Get a smaller waistline.

- Reduce cardiovascular risk factors.

- Get to a goal weight quickly—the size at which you look and feel most comfortable.

- Rapidly shed unwanted weight gained over a holiday or vacation.

- Break through frustrating weight loss plateaus.

- Stop the insane process of crash diets, fad diets, and yo-yo dieting.

- Get motivated to continue losing weight afterward, if you have a lot of weight to lose—and keep it off forever.

First, you and I are going to knock the extra weight off, to reveal the beautiful body that lies just beneath it. And we're going to do it fast—up to five pounds in five days. And up to twenty pounds the first month. Phase 1 of my plan is specially formulated to jump-start your metabolism and burn off excess weight, fast. I've also created a weekend plan that shows you how to indulge a bit more while still losing weight. My twenty-eight-day plan of super-delicious, healthy meals and recipes (including ready-made substitutions if you don't have time to cook) totals between 850 and 1,200 calories a day. It's based on the scientifically validated method of creating a "calorie deficit" that triggers weight loss, and in this case, using it to trigger steady weight loss over a twenty-eight-day period.

And second, in Phase 2, I'm going to ease you into a new food lifestyle you can enjoy for the rest of your life—a Mediterranean lifestyle not based on denial and self-torture over food, but on indulgence, pleasure, and pure satisfaction. It's a lifestyle that treats strict food rules as a bad idea—and considers snacks and treats an essential food group. This is a "gold standard" approach recommended by researchers and scientists around the world for maximizing your health and staying at a healthy weight.

This unique plan incorporates the most cutting-edge scientific breakthroughs on healthy weight loss. These breakthroughs have been discovered only recently, not by one or two self-appointed diet experts, but by multiple elite teams of the greatest doctors, scientists, and researchers around the world, working in the world's best universities and hospitals and research laboratories. They've made two stunning discoveries.

First, they've discovered a series of what I call Diet Booster Foods—specific "low-calorie-density" foods and ingredients that can actually accelerate the process of effective, healthy weight loss by supercharging your body to become a lean energy machine and manipulating your body's calorie-burning power. *The Pound a Day Diet* is built on a foundation of these Diet Booster Foods.

And second, these teams of doctors and scientists have identified an Ultimate Diet Pattern, a Mediterranean-style diet formula that the maintenance phase of this diet is based on. This is a pattern of eating you can and should follow for the rest of your life, which not only can help you reach your perfect weight, but can also:

- Keep the extra pounds from creeping back on.

- Lengthen your life.

- Improve your brain function.

- Defend you from chronic diseases.

- Fight certain cancers.

- Lower your risk of heart disease, high blood pressure, and elevated "bad" cholesterol levels.

- Protect you from diabetes.

- Keep away depression.

- Ward off Alzheimer's disease and Parkinson's disease.

- Ease rheumatoid arthritis.

- Improve your eye health.

- Reduce the risk of dental disease.

- Help you breathe better.

- Lead to healthier babies.

- Lead to improved fertility.

- Continue to boost your weight loss and management efforts, and, last but not least,

- Improve your sex life!

How's that for a highly excellent package of benefits? And it's all based on real science, not on hype. Believe it, it works for me!

I developed this diet plan with the guidance of a medical doctor and a registered dietitian. And I based the plan on the latest research on health, nutrition, and weight loss. My calorie-corrected, carb-corrected twenty-eight-day program will help you drop your extra weight. You'll start burning fat the first day. You'll learn how to easily avoid the stuff you don't need that can pack on the pounds, like excessive sugar, belly-busting portions, bad carbs, and bad fats. Trust me, though, you'll hardly miss them at all. I don't think you'll even know they're gone. I've included meal plans, shopping lists, and ready-made suggestions if you don't want to cook and are always on the go. And then we'll focus on a "maintenance" phase that you can put into action and enjoy for the rest of your life.

My sixty all-new recipes will inspire you to create delicious, healthy meals you'll enjoy—and that will help you keep the pounds off.

Finally, this plan is based on my own personal experience that fast, healthy weight loss is a terrific motivator. There are plenty of experts who argue that slow, gradual weight loss is best, and that approach may indeed work well for many people. But if you're like me, the inspiration and excitement you'll feel with rapid results will push you to achieve your ideal weight faster and stay there for good. This is a new philosophy that some experts are starting to embrace as a viable option for effective weight loss, and as an effective, highly motivating pathway to staying at your perfect weight.

Now let's get you started on your journey to fast, healthy weight loss!

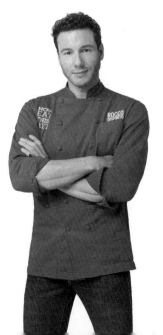

PART ONE

THE POUND A DAY DIET WEIGHT LOSS PRINCIPLES

CHAPTER 1

You Can Lose Weight in as Little as Five Days

YOU'RE probably wondering: What kind of diet is this, anyway?

This is a low-calorie, high-flavor diet, engineered for satisfaction, which is the crucial ingredient in any successful diet program.

How is this program different from other diets you've been on? Will you finally be able to lose weight and not gain it back?

If you've never been able to stay on a diet before, if you've never really made it to a healthy goal weight, or if you've been a chronic dieter for most of your life, this is a dramatically effective system that will change all that—and more. For one thing, you get to eat *delicious* food—in liberal amounts—as you drop pounds and inches.

This is a diet that keeps working for you as long as you need it—unlike most diets, which leave you wondering what to do after you've lost weight or get stalled by a frustrating plateau. As a result, you'll continue to burn fat, week after week—up to twenty pounds the very first month.

Here is why:

In Phase 1, you'll follow my specially formulated diet plan from Monday through Friday (or Sunday through Thursday, whatever best fits your lifestyle), then switch to the weekend plan, when you get to eat more food. All sorts of vegetables and fruits. Energizing carbs. A little wine on occasion, if that's what's right for you? Absolutely.

After the weekend, you simply return to the five-day weekday diet, then the weekend plan again. You keep following this sequence—five-day plan, weekend plan, five-day plan, weekend plan, and so forth, in a no-plateau beeline straight to your goal weight. In Phase 2, I'll outline a maintenance plan to help you keep the weight off and live a healthier lifestyle.

WHY YOU WILL SUCCEED THIS TIME!

For any diet to be successful, I believe the food has to taste great, be satisfying, and be nutritious, and the diet itself has to be uncomplicated *and* produce rapid results. Most important, it has to be livable, meaning that it instills a pattern of healthy eating so that you keep the weight off for good. These are the ingredients I consider essential for nutritious yet quick weight loss.

In today's immediate-gratification world, we want results fast—and that includes weight loss. Used to be, rapid weight loss was a no-no, but a new theory is emerging that the faster you take off weight, the longer you keep it off. In my experience, rapid weight loss is very psychologically motivating, so you're more likely to stick with a diet that gives you quick results.

Slow, gradual weight loss may in fact be best for some dieters, and this is the advice many experts have adhered to for years. But some experts are beginning to believe that healthy, faster weight loss based on a lower-calorie diet can be motivating and inspiring. I know that's true for me personally.

A team of researchers at the University of Melbourne in Australia is conducting an extraordinary ongoing pilot study with groups of dieters, using very-low-calorie liquid diet replacement meals. Their preliminary observations, reported in 2010, refuted the "slow, gradual weight loss is best" argument. "Surprisingly, and against current beliefs, this study shows rapid weight loss appears to be superior to gradual weight loss in achieving target weight," said University of Melbourne dietitian Katrina Purcell about the study, conducted on subjects weighing around 100 kilos (about 220 pounds), in a July 14, 2010, article in *AFP* (*Agence France-Presse*). Purcell, who is helping to conduct the study, told the *Herald Sun* (November 21,

2010): "Some 99.2% of nutritionists and dietitians say they recommend to their patients gradual weight loss over more rapid. However, there is absolutely no scientific evidence to support their claim."

Purcell speculated on the reason that fast weight loss was working: "Those people in the rapid group remained more motivated and were able to see the results coming. Those in the gradual group were more prone to becoming disenchanted." Importantly, she suggests, as I do, that weight loss be done under the supervision of a health care professional, like a dietitian.

"It is possible to lose weight, from [using] weird diets, to sensible eating, to exercise, but the most important thing is maintaining it," noted Timothy Gill, associate professor and principal research fellow at the University of Sydney's medical school's Boden Institute of Obesity, Nutrition, Exercise, and Eating Disorders, in a November 25, 2010, article in the *Australian Financial Review*. "Research coming out of Austin Hospital in Melbourne suggests we need a limited time for the weight loss phase before we enter into the weight maintenance phase. This has not become the accepted dogma, but there are suggestions it might work best."

Dr. David Carey, an Australian endocrinologist and obesity expert, has argued in favor of rapid weight loss, and told one journalist that he believes many dieters have a fixed window of opportunity to achieve success: "You have about six to nine months maximum—and the more you lose in that period, the more likely you are to keep it off," he observed. "The only reason that fast weight loss has traditionally been seen as bad is because to lose weight rapidly you usually need to undergo extreme measures. Many of these diets we hear about are completely unsustainable and difficult to stay on. Once people get to the end of them, if they can get to the end of them, they can't maintain their weight loss because they have no plan, eventually returning to their old eating habits" (*Sydney Telegraph*, November 21, 2010).

The Pound a Day Diet, by contrast, is based on real food and frequent healthy meals and includes a maintenance plan for the rest of your life that's grounded in real science.

On this diet you can get fast results—up to five pounds in just the first five days. How?

CALORIE CORRECTION

First, this is a calorie-reduced diet, or as I prefer to call it, a calorie-corrected diet. Quite simply, to lose weight you've got to correct and properly balance your calorie intake, first to reduce excess weight, and then to stay at your healthy weight. You do this through a combination of eating well and physical activity—but there are powerful shortcuts, which I'll tell you about shortly.

Calorie correction is extremely effective for getting lean quickly because you reset the body's machinery to put it on a course for healthy, sustained weight loss.

CARB CORRECTION

This diet is also a carb-corrected diet, where you'll switch from bad carbs to good carbs. This doesn't mean you need to give up bread or pasta—I could never do that to you! Instead, you'll learn about slow-burning carbs and how they can help you maintain your weight loss without feeling deprived.

The diet is designed to burn off fat fast, not by depriving you of food or sentencing you to bland diet food, but by recharging your metabolism and motivation so that you drop pounds, day in and day out.

MEDITERRANEAN STYLE: A DIET YOU CAN LIVE WITH AND LOSE ON FOR THE LONG TERM

The diet you're about to start is based on brand-new research into what works best over the short and long haul for rapid, safe, and satisfying weight loss—*a calorie-corrected, carb-corrected, Mediterranean diet pattern based on flavor and satisfaction*. The traditional Mediterranean diet is known as one of the healthiest diets around—and it's basically what I grew up on. I love this style of eating!

This sort of diet is based on vegetables, fruits, lean proteins, whole grains, and olive oil—plus an attitude that includes enjoying and savoring the experience of food and those with whom we break bread. **Whole-grain bread**, that is!

Of course, nothing kills your motivation to lose weight faster than a boring diet. So if you're tired of monotonous meals, you've found the right diet. Here you'll discover recipes and meal plans that are high on flavor and low on bad carbs, bad fats, and, very significantly, total calories. Healthful doesn't mean tasteless, either. A little variety is your ticket to sticking with your diet and getting the results you want. On this diet, I'll teach you how to prepare food—including a lot of your favorites.

This is a turbocharged weight loss program, and I've made it all simple for you. In fact, the recipes in this book are some of the simplest recipes I've ever come up with. This is real food, not "diet food"!

I'll show you simple tricks so you don't need to spend hours in the kitchen. I'll teach you how to eat sinfully without the sin!

I've learned many things on my weight loss journey and in creating this program, but there are three simple things I want you to remember as you begin your journey:

1. VEGGIES ARE A SECRET WEAPON

Vegetables like leafy greens have a high fiber or high water content but don't carry many calories. Eating veggies has many weight control advantages: They fill you up but supply very few calories. They're naturally diuretic—meaning they increase the flow of fluid from the body. (Water retention and bloating interfere with metabolism.) Green veggies are especially good to fill up on, and they include asparagus, cucumbers, spinach, lettuce (all varieties), mustard greens, parsley, collard greens, beet greens, turnip greens, kale, green beans, broccoli, dandelion greens, arugula, and watercress. Greens, in general, also supply generous doses of vitamins, minerals, antioxidants, phytochemicals, and fiber—all known to promote superb health. You can eat all the greens you want. And if you're not a veggie lover, don't worry…I'll give you some recipes that will convert you in no time.

2. LEAN PROTEIN ROCKS YOUR BODY

Proteins rev up your metabolism because the body requires more energy to process protein than carbohydrates. Protein also keeps you full and banishes food cravings. A study published in the journal *Obesity* in September 2011 demonstrated that protein intake promotes satiety (fullness); plus, it helps you retain lean body mass as you lose weight, which is critical for achieving the physique you want.

This diet provides enough protein to help burn belly fat, as well as visceral adipose tissue (VAT), a dangerous kind of fat that envelops organs and leads to disease and accelerated aging.

This diet also emphasizes foods that are high in protein, including eggs, chicken and turkey breast, fish, and even beef. Yes—you heard that right, beef. I love beef. I've been a sworn carnivore since birth. Taking beef away from me would make me quite depressed. Yes, I know that the antimeat police have declared that one person's steak has become every person's poison. But I believe that beef, in moderation and in the right portions, can be a great part of an overall healthy diet. Beef helps create stronger muscles, builds better bones, and boosts the growth of brain cells.

There's lots of variety when it comes to lean protein, and you can eat it in liberal quantities.

3. NUTRITIONAL BALANCE IS PARAMOUNT

Weight loss programs frequently get slammed, usually because they aren't always nutritious. I agree; this is true of a lot of diets. But I've observed that our everyday eating habits—not the diets we follow—are making us flabby and unhealthy. Most of us simply aren't eating nutritiously enough to get in even the basic daily requirements: vitamins, minerals, and fiber. So let's not just blame diets that don't work, let's blame our bad habits.

This diet is devised to provide a healthy combination of basic nutrients, including fiber, phytochemicals, antioxidants, vitamins, and minerals.

It's also based on three breakthrough diet insights from effective, scientifically based weight loss: calorie correction, carb correction, and the Mediterranean diet pattern, all of which you'll discover how to put into action.

When you put it all together, I believe this diet will change your life. Believe me, *you can do this*. My personal journey is proof that it works, if you stick with it.

The Bad News

- 72 percent of American men and 64 percent of American women are overweight or obese, with about one-third of American adults being obese.

- At least one-third of Americans are inactive, which raises health risks significantly.

- A shocking less than 5 percent of American adults perform the minimum recommendation of at least thirty minutes of physical activity each day, and only 8 percent of adolescents achieve their recommended goal of 60 minutes of daily physical activity.

- Obesity and overweight substantially increase the risks of hypertension, high blood cholesterol, type 2 diabetes, coronary heart disease, stroke, gallbladder disease, osteoarthritis, sleep apnea and respiratory problems, and several forms of cancer.

- Americans eat too many calories and too much saturated fat, added sugar, refined grain, and sodium—and too little potassium; dietary fiber; calcium; vitamin D; unsaturated fatty acids from oils, nuts, and seafood; and other important nutrients. These necessary nutrients are mostly found in vegetables, fruits, whole grains, and beans and legumes.

- People who eat out more often, especially at fast-food restaurants, are at higher risk for weight gain, overweight, and obesity, especially when they consume one or more fast-food meals per week.

- The food supply has changed radically over the past forty years. Average daily calories available per person in the marketplace have jumped by about 600, with the biggest jumps in the availability of added fats and oils, grains, milk and milk products, and caloric sweeteners.

- Many portion sizes also have increased. Research has shown that when larger portion sizes are served, people tend to consume more calories. In addition, strong evidence shows that portion size is associated with body weight, so that being served and consuming smaller portions are associated with weight loss.

Source: Centers for Disease Control and Prevention

- All these factors are things you can control. The power is in your hands!

- Losing just 5 to 10 percent of your current weight will help lower your risk of heart disease and many other medical disorders.

- You *can* lose weight, you *can* keep it off, and you *can* still enjoy versions of your favorite foods, as well as snacks and treats. In this book, I'll show you how.

I've spent the last several years devoted to healthy cooking that tastes amazing and helps you stay absurdly fit. As you probably know, my secret has been to rework America's favorite (and fattening) comfort foods into flavorful, low-calorie, low-fat, good-carb renditions that taste as good, if not better. That's what my **Now Eat This!** books are all about. Think fried chicken, pizza, macaroni and cheese, and chocolate ice cream. Yes, you can eat all that, if you prepare it using the techniques and recipes in my books.

I enjoy every molecule of food I eat. I eat frequently. In **The Pound a Day Diet** you'll enjoy all your meals and won't feel like you're on a diet at all. You'll lose the weight and keep it off, by following these fat loss principles:

- Your body needs good carbs, it needs good fats, and it needs lean protein. You should enjoy them in the right forms and the right amounts.

- Skip the gimmicks. Don't focus too much on high carb vs. low carb, or eliminating one type of food or another from your diet, or you'll miss the big picture.

- The big picture is this: You'll lose weight by using healthy calorie-corrected eating and regular physical activity to create a *calorie deficit*—and you'll maintain your weight loss by using the same tactics to keep in *calorie balance*.

- Both the quantity and the quality of the calories count. To lose weight, you've got to balance and upgrade your calories.

- A diet should focus what you *can* eat, and what you can eat *more of*, including low-calorie-density Diet Booster Foods like fruits and vegetables and whole grains.

- Healthy, rapid weight loss can be motivating and inspiring—but you need a maintenance plan for the rest of your life that combines healthy eating and physical activity.

- The perfect diet for you is the healthy one you can live with and enjoy, over the long haul, and is based on a pattern like the Mediterranean diet for overall health and weight control.

- A diet means lifelong pleasure.

- Don't deny yourself—indulge!

- Be flexible, but focus on working toward your target of a healthy weight.

- Snacks and treats are an essential food group.

The Skinny on Weight Loss Success

This diet experience was revolutionary for me. I'm pretty stupefied, dumbstruck, and shocked at how good it is. The results of the diet on my body have been unbelievable, and it was easy! I was on it for sixty-five days. I started at 146 pounds. At the end of seven days I was at 140 pounds. At the end of sixty-five days I was down to 124.2. And my body-fat percentage was as low as 21.2 percent.

My mother is a jazz musician who worked nights, so dinner and meals were not set in our family at all. She's a great mother, but we were often left to get our own food as teenagers. We were never exposed to home-cooked meals. It was a pizza pie or whatever we could grab. We were all healthy kids, we were athletes, and so it never really showed on us. We were thin and petite and basically got away with it for a long time.

As an adult, the thought of being able to plan a meal or sit down for one just was never an option. I'd often grab whatever was easiest, like two major handfuls of M&M's.

As I entered my forties I realized that being thin wasn't coming naturally to me anymore. I found that my body was holding on to whatever fat it could.

When I started this program Rocco said, "I have to teach you how to eat." Because I work sometimes eighteen to twenty hours a day and I wasn't sure 850 calories a day was enough. It seemed daunting. But when saw all the food I could eat in a week, I was surprised. I thought, "Can I eat all this food?" I didn't want to have to throw it in the trash.

Rocco said, "You're going to lose a pound a day." And I did. That was the first thing that shocked me. The next thing that shocked me was that it stuck. I felt amazing the first month, and after that I felt phenomenal.

The most amazing thing that has happened to me is I am actually cooking now. My friends and family simply cannot fathom the fact that I am in the kitchen.

I'm completely transformed. My body is so different now. The only bone I have to pick with Rocco is that my clothes are way too big on me now!

—Suzanne

QUICK START INSTRUCTIONS

ROCCO'S SEVEN INSTANT ACTION TIPS TO BLAST EXTRA WEIGHT OFF

If you're like I was, and are one of the millions of Americans who are obese or are overweight by twenty, thirty, or more pounds, not moving enough and consuming 1,000 calories or more per day more than you should be, here's a quick checklist of things you can do right now to start getting on the fast track toward your healthy weight—before you even start reading the rest of this book!

Put all these tips together, put them into action, and watch the weight melt right off your beautiful, rock-star body. These are the things I do to stay at a perfect, great-feeling weight. You can do it!

1. **Run, don't walk, to your doctor for a full physical and a medical opinion** *on your weight loss goals and strategies, including those you'll learn in this book.*

2. **Don't starve yourself or skip meals. Instead, adopt a delicious new food lifestyle you can enjoy for the rest of your life, based on**

whole foods, healthy eating patterns, and total pleasure. *Don't go on unproven, non–medically supervised fad diets, crash diets, detoxes, diet pills, cleanses, or colonics if you're looking for healthy, sustainable weight loss. In most cases the weight will bounce right back on.*

3. Focus on foods you should enjoy. Indulge in good carbs from veggies and whole grains, and good fats like omega-3s from fish; and accelerate your weight loss with Diet Booster Foods like veggies, fruits, whole grains, beans and legumes, and broth-based soups. *Dial way down the sodium, refined carbs, processed foods, added sugars and saturated fat, and junky snacks. That's the Rocco-style, Mediterranean-style Ultimate Diet Pattern, and it's as close to a perfect model diet for weight loss and overall health as you'll find.*

4. Correct your portion sizes by downsizing them by one-fourth, one-third, or even one-half. *This sounds very simple and painfully obvious, but it's absolutely critical. You need to realize that most American food portion sizes are designed for wild beasts, not people. Correct, smaller portion sizes are what help keep people like the Italians and French very healthy and slim, and you should eat these smaller portions, too.* By correcting your portion sizes and increasing your physical activity, you can easily cut 500 to over 1,000 calories a day, and that's the formula you need to blast off the fat.

5. Make water your main beverage. *Forget the sugary beverages— sugary sweet teas, fruit drinks, and sodas. They're history, they're totally passé. If you think you can't live without them, think again. I predict you'll hardly remember them in a few days. Reach instead for water, ice water, or water with a lemon or lime twist.* It's all you'll ever need as your main drink, *and it's all you'll ever need to give your family—period, end of story.*

6. Shake your butt. Insist on treating yourself to a nonnegotiable, soul-refreshing reward of at least an hour of moderate-to-intense physical activity on most days of the week. *Power-walking counts, as long as it's vigorous, and so do shorter bursts of vigorous*

physical activity spread through the day. You can burn off 500 calories a day or more this way.

7. Enjoy and indulge. *Savor every morsel of food you eat. Food is fun, food is family, and food is joy. Smile, and say this three times slowly:* Food...is...love!

The Skinny on Weight Loss Success

I lost six and a half to seven pounds in seven days. It felt great to lose weight that quickly, but it also felt good to know that my body had reached a new "set point"—the weight hasn't come back. This diet took real body weight off, not just water weight.

My lifestyle is busy and hectic. I'm constantly on the go, eating out a lot—restaurant and takeout food that is calorie dense. Over the years, I've been on every kind of diet, and nothing has tasted as good as Rocco's Pound a Day Diet, or worked as well. You'll experience a change in the way you look at food, and begin to understand that you can do something to make a lifestyle change forever.

That's what's great about what Rocco does. He takes the foods we've been eating forever and makes them accessible. He makes them delicious. He makes them lower in calories, lower in fat, and lets us eat the things we like.

I used to eat a few big meals a day, and didn't really understand that all calories aren't created equal. I didn't understand that until I met Rocco. He taught me the importance of eating a lot of meals over the course of a day and making them smaller. Smaller meals all day long, eating within a half hour of waking up, and eating big, filling things that have fewer calories.

The food on this diet is delicious. The gazpacho was as good as anything I've had at Le Cirque! I didn't know that gazpacho could be low-calorie and taste like something you get in a restaurant. I think taste has a lot to do with how you stay on a diet. Because this food tastes so good, it's easier to stay on.

This is a lifestyle change based on your making a better series of choices. And it works!

—Brendan

CHAPTER 2

Calorie Correction and the Secret of Diet Booster Foods

I'LL bet you gained weight like I did—completely by accident.

Slowly but surely, over time, as you worked hard at your job, shuttled your kids to school and soccer practice, relaxed with your family and friends, ate out at restaurants, grabbed fast food from time to time, and worked harder and harder, you noticed it happening, but really gradually.

Your pants started getting tighter.

You got more winded when you raced up the stairs.

Clothes started not fitting you. You started moving and exercising more slowly, and less and less often.

Then, one day…WHAM-O!…Somehow you wound up on a scale and you noticed you'd put on ten pounds! Or twenty! Or even thirty! Maybe you thought what I did—"Oh, no, how did this happen!"

That's just what happened to me.

I was a young chef, and a successful one at that. I'd won awards, garnered glowing reviews, and appeared on magazine covers. I had two hot restaurants, and fantastic food was all around me.

And I started porking out on all that wonderful food. I got fat really slowly. I didn't even notice. Nobody told me, "Hey, you need to lose weight!" We're all used to fat chefs. We're used to chefs being jolly and round and robust. Being chubby is part of the job. I didn't care about healthy eating or dieting.

When I had my own restaurant, I wasn't eating so much as a reward or from stress or emotional pressure; I was eating as a duty to my customers! I had to taste the food I made and I had to constantly audit and evaluate the menu. It was just part of my job.

At the end of each night I would sit at table 21 and I would order five or six of the dishes. I'd give my kitchen staff extensive notes on the experience, and try to make improvements for the next day. And if there was an incredibly perfect foie gras, or bluefin tuna that came in with tremendous belly fat, or some great pork belly, of course I had to try it. Hey, it's just what chefs do! It was part of embracing and participating in this search for great flavor. And nothing got in my way.

I always say the difference between a good chef and a great chef is how often they eat their own food. It's true. You don't know if the architecture of your dish is coming out right unless you taste it and eat the whole thing. You can't just take a bite. So every night, it would happen. I stuffed my belly with succulent food. There would always be a lot of wine, because we were doing wine pairings with the sommelier. I was eating thousands of calories a day more than my body needed.

Overeating became a ritual for me. It was pleasurable and it was crucial for my work. I also had to go out to other restaurants and taste the food of the new chefs, and constantly do food research. I was oblivious to the fact that this routine was causing me to pack on the pounds.

Before I knew it, I was close to a thirty-eight-inch waist, and I was topping out at nearly 220 pounds. I was approaching thirty-seven years old.

I was old enough to start to feel the impact. And it scared me a little bit. I realized you have to be healthy to be successful at anything. I wasn't able to stand up easily; I didn't have the endurance I'd had when I was in my twenties. It started affecting my work—I could see that it hampered my ability to cook with the right amount of energy.

I got worried. Then my doctor gave me some bad news about my cholesterol, body fat, and blood pressure. He urgently requested that I reassess my lifestyle. He gave me a choice. He said, "You can take these three medicines, or you can change your diet and exercise."

Right around that time, surprisingly, I got out of the day-to-day restaurant business—something I never expected to happen. I realized, "Oh, I don't have a restaurant to go to tomorrow; maybe I should go to the gym!" I called up my old trainer, dabbled more intensely. I started doing triathlons and watching what I ate. I realized the importance of watching my calories. I began experimenting in the kitchen to create lower-calorie, healthy dishes that were still delicious.

As I steadily lost the extra weight through smarter, healthier eating and exercise, I went from an extra-large size, down to a large size, down to a medium. People started telling me, "You look younger!" My doctor said, "You're healthier! Your cholesterol is down. How did you do it?" Now I'm down to a thirty-three or thirty-four-inch waist and my weight is in the 180s, with a lot more lean muscle, which is optimal for me.

I started getting focused on losing weight because I wanted to get healthy, and now I see that getting yourself to the commitment is the hard part. Once you're committed from your heart to your brain to your whole body, it's a lot easier. The time between the moment when you recognize you have an issue and the day you take action is the challenge.

It's like when you haven't seen someone in ten years and they say, "Wow, you used to be so thin! What happened?" And you think, "I'm fat? I didn't know I was fat! No one told me I was fat! Oh my God, let me go weigh myself. I weighed 170, now I'm 190! I can't believe it!" The time between that moment and the moment you say to yourself, "I'm really going to do something about it," really is the hardest part of losing weight. The hardest part is getting to that moment when you commit to eating right and going to the gym and not debating with yourself whether you really will.

I don't think gaining the weight was our fault. We live in an obesogenic environment, where junk food, beast-sized portions, unhealthy snacks, and really bad food choices are all around us, every single day, all the time. Part of our problem with obesity is that we live in a minimum-required culture. It's a culture of extreme convenience where everything is brought to you. You don't have to go out and hunt and gather food, the way our bodies were designed to do by Mother Nature. Shopping and cooking are all drive-thru, remote control, takeout, delivery, and an extremely sedentary lifestyle that results in no calories burned.

The main reason you and I got fat was that we slowly lost control of the simple formula that governs our weight: We started taking in more calories than we burned off over time, over the course of days, weeks, and months. It all averaged out to a calorie surplus, and Mother Nature responded by sticking a big spare tire of fat on our body. As for me, I was probably scarfing down 1,000 too many calories per day on average, and every one of those pesky creatures turned into pure body chunk.

CALORIES COUNT

There's no way around it—calories count. Sure, interesting research may pop up in the media about how your weight may be influenced by your heredity or by this hormone or that food ingredient, but the big picture is all about calories. As the 2010 Dietary Guidelines for Americans put it, "People who are most successful at losing weight and keeping it off do so through continued attention to calorie balance." And the quality of calories counts, too.

The first step in blasting off the fat is figuring out where your weight is right now. Step two is figuring out where you want to be and should be. And step three is adjusting and rebalancing your calorie formula to get you there. The program in Phase 1 of my diet is already calorie corrected to help you reach your goal weight quickly. But once you have reached your goal, you'll need to adjust your daily calorie count to help you keep the weight off. I'll cover all this in Phase 2 of the plan.

It's simpler than you think. If you correct your personal calorie formula, the weight will fall off and stay off. I like to call this calorie correction, and it's one of the principles of my program. The great news is that you can do it. You can correct your calorie count to blast the extra weight off your body and keep it off. Absolutely. And you and I will make it a delicious journey.

More good news: When you lose unhealthy extra weight, you can significantly improve the way you feel every day, your energy level, your happiness, your sex life, your productivity, and your protection against a host of health risks, like heart disease, stroke, high blood pressure, various cancers, sleep apnea, type 2 diabetes, arthritis, osteoporosis, and premature death.

I know you want to get rid of the fat now.

That's how I felt when I was thirty pounds overweight—something I hate to admit.

I know you're asking yourself: "Am I capable of doing this, of getting down to a healthy and normal weight, of breaking my fat cycle [not talking about your bike here], and of losing so much flab I can actually fit into the ridiculously small sizes my spouse or significant other fantasizes about? And if so, how much weight can I drop—and how fast?"

Let's discuss ways to arrive at a healthy goal weight, and start by seeing how much you've got to lose.

> *If you're one to ten pounds overweight: If you're not more than ten pounds overweight, this diet is a great way to reach your goal in roughly two to ten days. And if you follow the maintenance plan in Phase 2 of the diet, you will keep it off.*
>
> *If you're eleven to twenty pounds overweight: If you fit into this category, it could take you as little as one month—maybe less—to lose the weight. And you may lose even more. Lucky you. This diet is designed to help you lose up to one pound a day, so it's relatively easy to reach your goal quickly.*
>
> *If you're twenty-one to fifty pounds overweight: If you have this much to lose, don't despair. It could take you a little longer to lose it—two months or so. Chances are, you're hanging on to a lot of water weight. People with a lot of weight to lose tend to retain more fluid than those who aren't so overweight. So you might end up losing weight faster than you ever imagined possible.*
>
> *If you're more than fifty pounds overweight: By following this diet, you'll probably lose weight rapidly at first; then your weight loss may slow down slightly. However, you could lose a significant amount of weight in about three months.*

Portion Explosion from the 1980s to the 2000s

Is it any wonder that America has put on tons of weight?

The food and restaurant industries have slowly exploded the average portion sizes of the foods we eat over the last few decades. I'm surprised we all don't weigh 300 pounds each by now:

CALORIES IN A TYPICAL SERVING

	1980s	2000s
Bagel	140	350
Cheeseburger	333	590
Spaghetti and meatballs	500	1,025
French fries	210	610
Soft drink	85	250
Turkey sandwich	320	820
Muffin	210	500
Pepperoni pizza	500	850
Caesar salad	390	790
Popcorn	270	630
Cheesecake	260	640
Chocolate chip cookie	55	275
Chicken stir-fry	435	865

Source: National Institutes of Health

CREATE A FAT-BLASTING CALORIE DEFICIT

There is a simple formula to losing weight, and it has nothing to do with pills, potions, or cutting out entire food groups. The formula is called a calorie deficit. A calorie deficit, quite simply, means you consume fewer calories in the form of food and beverages than you burn off in physical activity.

This diet is based on the rule of thumb that a deficit of 3,500 calories can result in a pound of fat loss. This guideline has been widely used by experts and health authorities like the National Institutes of Health, the American Dietetic Association, and the United Kingdom's National Health Service. But it is important to remember that this is only a guideline, and some experts consider it an oversimplification, as it doesn't properly account for individual differences, the effects of physical activity, and the body's adaptive mechanisms (see page 283).

In other words, your mileage may vary! But there's one thing the experts agree on: A calorie deficit over time will result in weight loss. And there are three ways to create a calorie deficit—eat fewer calories, do more physical activity, or combine the two.

For example, suppose you're a thirty-five-year-old woman, overweight because you consume a typical American diet of well over 3,000 calories a day and are only moderately physically active. According to the chart on page 225, you should be eating and drinking 2,000 calories to be in "calorie balance" and stay at a normal healthy weight. The excess calories you consume every day accumulate and settle on your body as extra weight.

While the "3,500 calories = 1 pound of fat loss" formula is only a rough guideline, and your mileage (and tonnage) may vary according to your sex, body type, age, starting weight, and other factors, here's how you can put the calorie deficit formula into action to lose weight:

Example 1

45 minutes of brisk walking (3.5 mph)
= 259 calories burned off per day
Plain coffee instead of large vanilla latte
= 241 fewer calories consumed per day
Creates:
500-calorie deficit per day, or about a pound a week off

Example 2

90 minutes of very brisk walking (4.0 mph)
= 681 calories burned off per day
Consuming nutritionally balanced 850 calories per day instead of
3,700 calories per day = 2,850 less calories consumed per day
Creates:
3,531-calorie deficit per day, or up to a pound a day off

In July 2012, the *New York Times* published an interview with one of the world's greatest experts on obesity and weight loss, Dr. Jules Hirsch, emeritus professor and physician-in-chief emeritus at Rockefeller University. Dr. Hirsch has been studying obesity for nearly sixty years, and he dismisses the idea that tinkering with different food types or tweaking fat or carbohydrate percentages is the key to weight loss. Instead, he said, it really all does boil down to calories.

According to Dr. Hirsch, "Perhaps the most important illusion is the belief that a calorie is not a calorie but depends on how much carbohydrates a person eats. There is an inflexible law of physics—energy taken into the body in the form of calories must exactly equal the number of calories leaving the system when fat storage is unchanged. Calories leave the system when food is used to fuel the body. To lower fat content—reduce obesity— one must reduce calories taken in, or increase the output by increasing activity, or both. This is true whether calories come from pumpkins or peanuts or pâté de foie gras. To believe otherwise is to believe we can find a really good perpetual motion machine to solve our energy problems. It won't work, and neither will changing the source of calories permit us to disobey the laws of science."

When the interviewer asked him what he would tell someone who wants to lose weight, the wise doctor replied, "I would have them eat a lower-calorie diet. They should eat whatever they normally eat, but eat less. You must carefully measure this. Eat as little as you can get away with, and try to exercise more."

There you have it. After sixty years of failed diet fads, weight loss books, and billions of dollars of pills and shakes, Dr. Hirsch boils it all down to the simplest of formulas for weight loss.

I've used this formula in the creation of my program, but I've added one crucial tweak: ***Enjoy yourself***. As a chef and someone who has lost weight and kept it off, I know that calorie correction can work only if you don't feel deprived by the diet.

That's why I've created all-new, delicious low-calorie recipes to help you lose the weight—while you enjoy the food!

LOW-CALORIE
DIET BOOSTER FOODS

My belly is the boss of how much I eat.

My belly likes to feel full.

And I obey my belly.

But I've discovered a secret to getting there, to making my belly happy. It's a secret that has been uncovered by some of the greatest nutrition scientists and researchers on the planet. And it can totally transform your body. The secret to eating a calorie-corrected diet is *low-calorie-density foods*.

The experts call it the concept of food energy density, or calorie density.

I call it the Secret of Diet Booster Foods, or low-calorie-density foods.

What if there were certain foods that could actually boost your chances of succeeding on a diet?

There actually are such foods, and if you enjoy them the right way, they can help you take the pounds off your body faster. They can accelerate the progress of your diet.

The technical term for them is low-calorie-density or low-energy-density foods, and their importance to weight control was first publicized by Dr. Barbara J. Rolls, a professor at Pennsylvania State University.

Calorie density, quite simply, is the number of calories per a certain weight of food:

- Foods that are processed or refined or have added sugars are higher-calorie-density foods, which is what you want much less of—because they help you put on weight and sabotage your weight control efforts.

- Foods with more fiber and water content, which also tend to be whole foods with more healthy nutrients, are lower-calorie-density foods, which is what you want more of—*because they help you lose weight. I call them Diet Booster Foods.*

In April 2012, a major report was published in the *Journal of the Academy of Nutrition and Dietetics* that found that consuming a diet that is relatively low in calorie density improves weight loss and weight maintenance. The study's lead investigator, Rafael Perez-Escamilla, PhD, of Yale University, said that the study supports the need to "consume such foods as fruits, vegetables, whole grains, and lean animal protein sources," which are usually lower in calorie density, and eat less total fat, saturated fat, and added sugars, which increase the calorie density of foods. Many people think that eating high-calorie foods will make them feel full. However, studies of food consumption in recent years have suggested that the *volume* of food, not calories, makes people feel full. And that's a huge insight to help you lose weight.

When you read reports of experts quibbling over this or that percentage of protein, fat, or carbs in a diet, don't forget this major insight that you can put into action right now to start losing weight fast—a mega-insight that many of the best experts agree on. As researchers at the Centers for Disease Control and Prevention put it: "Significant weight loss can occur when advice to increase intake of fruits and vegetables is coupled with advice to reduce energy intake [calories]."

At Pennsylvania State University, Professor Barbara Rolls and her colleagues and other researchers have conducted some fascinating experiments with different foods and beverages that have found that significant weight loss can occur when people combine two simple, fundamental steps: #1: Control the overall number of calories they eat, and #2: Enjoy more Diet Booster Foods, like fruits and vegetables.

In one amazing study, people were offered as much food as they wanted for five days from two alternating eating patterns. Eating pattern #1 was based on high-calorie-density foods, and eating pattern #2 was based on lower-calorie-density foods—in other words, more Diet Booster Foods. The researchers made a stunning discovery: When they followed pattern #2, the participants felt full **on half the calories** (1,570 calories) they needed to feel full on pattern #1 (3,000 calories)!

Just think of how much weight you could lose, and how fast, if you put this simple secret to work!

Believe it or not, air can influence your weight, too. Professor Rolls conducted a four-week study involving twenty-eight men and a test of the filling power of yogurt milk shakes. The shakes were given to the men thirty minutes before lunch on three different days. The shakes came in three sizes: 300 milliliters, 450 milliliters, and 600 milliliters. Each had the same number of calories; the larger volumes were created by incorporating air into the drinks. Guess what? Participants consumed 12 percent fewer calories at lunch after drinking the 600-milliliter milk shake, and reported greater feelings of fullness after drinking the 450-milliliter milk shake or the 600-milliliter milk shake than after the 300-milliliter shake.

In another four-week study, Professor Rolls and her colleagues found that eating a bowl of soup before lunch (they chose chicken-rice) significantly increased the feeling of fullness, reduced the participants' hunger, and significantly reduced the number of calories consumed at lunch. And another study found that adding Diet Booster Foods like carrots and spinach to meals, but keeping the same number of calories, enhanced the feeling of being full, if at least 200 grams of vegetables were added. It turns out that the calorie density of any eating pattern can be lowered simply by adding fruits and vegetables.

All foods fall into one of three categories:

- **High-calorie-density foods:** like cookies, crackers, butter, bacon, spareribs, potato chips, and many processed foods with added sugars. *Minimize the amounts of these foods and the frequency with which you eat them.*

- **Medium-calorie-density foods:** like bagels, dried fruits, thin-crust cheese pizza, and premium ice cream. *Enjoy on occasion, in moderate amounts.*

- **Diet Booster Foods lower in calorie density:** like most fruits and vegetables, fat-free yogurt, broth-based soups, cooked whole grains like oatmeal, beans, and modest portions of lean proteins like meat and fish. *Enjoy and indulge; base your diet on a foundation of these types of foods.*

The Secret of How Diet Booster Foods Work

- You stop eating when you feel full, but feeling full is based on the volume of food you eat, not necessarily on the calories contained in the food.

- Water and fiber are key ingredients that increase a food's volume and reduce its calories per food weight. Most fruits and vegetables are perfect examples of Diet Booster Foods, because they're high in both water and fiber, and low in calories per food weight.

- If you eat Diet Booster Foods, which are low-calorie-density foods, or foods with low calories per food weight, *you can feel full with fewer calories, and stop eating sooner.*

- Switching in more Diet Booster Foods to your diet can accelerate the success of your healthy eating plan and help you lose weight faster.

If you want to begin making Diet Booster Foods blast off the weight immediately, below are some guidelines that will help you get started now—and make a big difference in your diet:

1. *Build lots of fruits and vegetables into your meals, like spinach, cruciferous vegetables such as broccoli and cauliflower, peppers, zucchini, tomatoes, citrus fruits, and melons, to name just a few. Add them into your omelets, lasagna, chili, soups, and other hot dishes. Broth-based soups, which are also low in calorie density, are filling, low-calorie food choices. Also choose these foods as snacks and appetizers.*

2. *Round out meals by adding whole grains, beans and legumes, and correct portions of lean meat and fish. Using lower-fat meat and cheese or simply using less of the higher-saturated-fat ingredients can reduce the unhealthy fat content.*

3. *Minimize your consumption of high-calorie-density choices like fried foods, including fried vegetables; refined grains; dairy foods that are not reduced in fat; fatty cuts of meat; crackers; cookies; chips; croissants; margarine; and bacon. Eat them only occasionally, in small portions.*

4. *Make healthy foods like nuts and olives, which have good amounts of healthy polyunsaturated and monounsaturated fatty acids, part of your diet—as long as you eat them in moderate portions.*

Sources: CDC, author's research

When you add up all these tips, the weight will melt off. It's that simple.

Are you tired of diets that tell you what **not** to eat?

Well, I've got great news for you.

One of the keys to healthy, effective, fast weight loss is for you to **eat more**—eat more Diet Booster Foods.

It totally works for me and I bet it will for you, too.

In addition to calorie correction and Diet Booster Foods, let's put another fantastic weight loss secret to work for you—the power of slow carbs.

The Skinny on Weight Loss Success

When I started this diet, I was trying to lose about five pounds in a week. I started out at 121 pounds and by the end of seven days I was at 115, so I lost 6 pounds in a week!

The diet was very easy because I was never hungry. There was always something every couple of hours for me to eat that was really filling. I didn't have all those impulses to eat bad food. I looked forward to the apples and cheese every day, and also the chocolate smoothie in the morning, which was great! There was enough snacking and frequency of eating. And it wasn't just lettuce and cucumbers; it was actually food I enjoyed. I felt completely satisfied, and I was losing about a pound a day.

Once I hit my goal, I felt like I knew what foods I could eat to maintain the weight. My mind-set had changed. Also, when you change your lifestyle and you eat healthier foods, it makes a difference in your energy. Now I feel like I have more energy.

The whole experience was great!

—Vicki

CHAPTER 3

Carb Correction and the Fat-Blasting Power of Slow Carbs

NOT long ago, I made a simple switch that changed my life.

And it helped knock thirty pounds off my body.

I decided to switch to slow carbs. If you replace the simple carbohydrates in your diet with slow-burning complex carbohydrates—a change I call carb correction—you'll discover one of the most powerful secrets for effective weight loss and overall health.

For years, I loved to indulge in fairly unlimited amounts of white bread, white pasta, white rice, and, of course, added sugars, which are built into a gazillion American foods and beverages that are all around us.

Looking for a guy to serve hard time in a spaghetti factory?

That was me.

Need some help polishing off a stack of old-fashioned pancakes, bagels with cream cheese, bread and butter, or Kaiser rolls?

I was your man.

Back up the white flour truck and pour it all over me, I figured. Bring it on!

Would you like to know what the #1 ranking source of calories among Americans is, ahead of soda, burgers, potato chips, and pizza? It's grain-based desserts. Cake, cookies, pie, cobbler, sweet rolls, pastries, and donuts. That one group of foods puts more calories on our bodies than any other, and I used to eat them indiscriminately.

No wonder I was packing so much extra freight on my belly!

What I didn't fully realize then was that most of these high-calorie foods had had a lot of the nutrition stripped out of them by the Great American Food Processing Machine. And worse, because they were so heavily processed and had such a high glycemic index, they were, over time, spiking my blood sugar and triggering a vicious cycle of spikes, crashes, and cravings that helped make me fat.

Then, as I researched the science of losing weight and the art of creating great food to make it happen, I discovered the fat-blasting power of slow-burning carbs.

Have no fear. I will not be suggesting that you eliminate carbs from your life. You've **got** to have carbs in your diet.

Carb is not a four-letter word!

You've just got to choose the good carbs.

Carbohydrates, it turns out, actually play a role in fat burning, as long as you choose the right types of carbohydrates. This is where carbohydrate choice becomes all-important to your weight loss success.

Slow-burning carbs are foods like whole grains and beans that are rich in complex carbohydrates. They're a critical aid to help you to lose weight.

But get this—less than 5 percent of Americans eat the minimum recommended amount of whole grains! Are you one of them? Come on, fess up! I've been there myself.

Eaten in the right patterns and amounts, and especially if you eat them in place of less healthy foods, slow-burning carbs can help you feel less hungry between meals, feel fuller faster, and eat less overall. The authors of the US government's 2010 Dietary Guidelines for Americans put it well when they recommended: "When choosing carbohydrates, Americans should emphasize naturally occurring carbohydrates, such as those found in whole grains, beans and peas, vegetables, and fruits, especially those high in dietary fiber, while limiting refined grains and intake of foods with added sugars."

Let's take whole grains, for example. Whole grains, or foods made from them, contain all the essential parts and nutrients of the whole original grain seed. This means that 100 percent of the original kernel—all of the bran, germ, and endosperm—is present in what you eat:

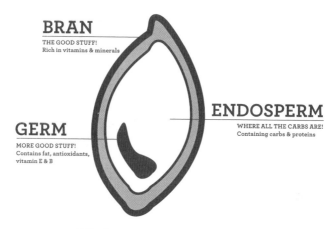

BRAN
THE GOOD STUFF!
Rich in vitamins & minerals

ENDOSPERM
WHERE ALL THE CARBS ARE!
Containing carbs & proteins

GERM
MORE GOOD STUFF!
Contains fat, antioxidants,
vitamin E & B

GRAIN ANATOMY

TO LOSE WEIGHT, GET THE WHOLE STUFF!

White bread, white rice, and other refined grains have had the germ and bran of the grain stripped out. Big mistake! That's where a lot of the nutrition and the fat-blasting power of whole grains are. And too many refined grains and simple carbohydrates can lead to weight gain because the body processes them less efficiently than complex carbs like beans and whole grains.

Instead of refined grains and simple carbs, you should choose whole-grain cereals and breads as part of your weight loss plan.

Why should you eat whole grains to lose weight?

Let us count the ways:

1. *Whole grains are rich in nutrients and bioactive components like iron, magnesium, selenium, B vitamins, and dietary fiber, plus slowly digestible energy, phytochemicals, and antioxidants.*

2. *Many whole-grain dishes, especially those cooked and served with water, like brown rice and oatmeal, are lower in calorie density and therefore qualify as Diet Booster Foods.*

3. *A number of studies have found that adults who eat more whole grains, especially those higher in dietary fiber, have* **lower body weight, less weight gain, and smaller waist size** *compared to adults who eat less whole grains.*

4. *A team of Dutch researchers studied 4,000 adults ages fifty-five to sixty-nine and found that higher whole-grain consumption was associated with lower BMI (body mass index) and a* **lower risk of overweight and obesity** (European Journal of Clinical Nutrition, *January 2009).*

5. *In a clinical study at Penn State, researchers put fifty obese adults on a lower-calorie diet for twelve weeks, during which time half the group was asked to eat all their grains as whole grains, and the other half was advised to avoid whole-grain foods. The whole-grain group saw a significantly greater* **decrease in abdominal fat** (American Journal of Clinical Nutrition, *January 2008).*

6. *UK researchers reviewed the stats on nearly 120,000 subjects and found that a higher intake of whole grains (about three servings a day) was associated with* **lower BMI and less abdominal fat** (Public Health Nutrition, *November 16, 2007).*

7. *Researchers at the University of Rhode Island, in a six-month study, found that whole-grain cereals helped 180 overweight adults* **lose weight** *while increasing their consumption of essential nutrients* (Journal of the American Dietetic Association, *September 2006).*

8. *A study of the health records of 72,000 men found that those who ate 40 grams of whole grains per day (like just one cup of cooked oatmeal or two slices of whole-wheat bread)* **cut middle-age weight gain by up to 3.5 pounds** (American Journal of Clinical Nutrition, *November 2004).*

9. *Eating whole grains has been associated not only with losing weight but also with a lower risk of developing type 2 diabetes, cardiovascular diseases, and cancer.*

10. *If that's not enough, eating whole grains has also been associated with reduced risk of asthma, healthier carotid arteries, reduction of inflammatory disease risk, healthier blood pressure levels, less gum disease, and less tooth loss.*

Sources: wholegrainscouncil.org, author's research

WHOLE GRAINS MAY ACT AS AN APPETITE SUPPRESSANT

Exactly how do whole grains help you lose weight?

Studies have revealed several properties of whole-grain foods and how the body responds to them. For example: They have a lower calorie density than many other foods. They also make you feel fuller and more satisfied, thereby acting as an appetite suppressant. And they have a lower glycemic index—they tend to raise blood sugar levels less. These are all likely reasons why whole grains contribute to weight loss.

Carbohydrates are classified as either simple or complex. Simple carbohydrates are found in candies, syrups, many fruits and fruit juices, and processed foods; complex carbohydrates are found in whole grains, beans, and vegetables. Whole grains are rich in health-promoting fiber as well.

Dietary fiber is the edible parts of plants, or similar carbohydrates that resist digestion and absorption in the small intestine. And recently, scientists have identified **six potential weight loss "activator" fibers** that are contained in various whole-grain and vegetable products. Here they are, along with their possible benefits:

1. *Arabinoxylan (AX): (don't try to say that with a mouthful of whole grains!): a fiber found in whole grains that helps control body weight, as well as blood sugar.*

2. *Inulin: a fiber in foods like onions, garlic, artichokes, and bananas that suppresses appetite.*

3. *Beta-glucan: a fiber in foods like whole-grain oats and barley that helps with blood sugar control and decreases unhealthy cholesterol in the body.*

4. **Pectin:** *a fiber found in lots of fruits and veggies, like apples, plums, grapes, bananas, blackberries, cranberries, green beans, legumes, squash, and sweet potatoes, that protects against obesity.*

5. **Cellulose:** *a fiber found in carrots, Brussels sprouts, cabbage, yams, alfalfa, lima beans, apricots, peas, and grapes that is very filling and helps you eat fewer calories overall.*

6. **Resistant starch:** *a type of carbohydrate that is not completely absorbed in the small intestine as other foods are, and bypasses the fate of most carbs, which can get deposited as body fat if you eat more than you can burn off. Instead, resistant starch migrates to the large intestine, where it escorts fats and calories out of the body. Top sources of resistant starch include beans (kidney, pinto, black, garbanzo, and so forth), bananas (slightly green), yams, sweet potatoes, potatoes, and whole grains like barley and brown rice.*

TIPS TO BOOST YOUR WHOLE GRAINS AND SLOW CARBS

To get a 100 percent whole-grain food, look for the first ingredient listed on the package to use the word **whole**. Be aware that "multigrain," "seven-grain," "wheat," and other kinds of bread are often not fully whole-grain, so be sure to check that ingredient list and make sure a "whole" grain is listed first. For foods with multiple whole-grain ingredients, they should appear near the beginning of the ingredient list. These foods and ingredients, when eaten in a form including the bran, germ, and endosperm, are examples of generally accepted whole-grain foods and flours:

- amaranth*
- barley
- buckwheat*
- corn, including whole cornmeal and popcorn*
- millet*
- oats, including oatmeal**
- quinoa*
- rice, both brown rice and colored rice*

- rye
- sorghum (also called milo)*
- teff*
- triticale
- wheat, including varieties such as spelt, emmer, farro, einkorn, Kamut, durum, and forms such as bulgur, cracked wheat, and wheat berries
- wild rice*

There are many ways to introduce more whole grains to your diet. Here are just a few of the methods I've found of powering up the whole grains:

- **Wake up with whole grains.** Instead of bacon and sausage or donuts for breakfast every morning, switch over to a bowl of oatmeal, lightly sweetened with fruit, stevia, or a little sugar. Look for simple old-fashioned oats and steer clear of the sugar-filled flavored packets. Or switch to a low-sugar or unsweetened cold whole-grain cereal.

- **For sandwiches, switch from white bread to whole-grain bread.** Remember that there are many breads out there with names like *multigrain*, *seven-grain*, and *wheat*, but many of them are not really whole grain. Check the ingredient list and make sure the first ingredient has the word *whole* in it, as in *whole wheat*.

- **Experiment with whole grains you haven't tried much,** like brown rice, bulgur, wheat berries, millet, or hulled barley, as part of your dinner.

- **Switch to whole-grain pasta.** It's heartier, chewier, and much better for you than pastas based on refined grains. Check the ingredient list and make sure the first ingredient has the word *whole* in it.

Note: Whole wheat is one kind of whole grain, so all whole wheat is whole grain, but not all whole grain is whole wheat.
* If you're concerned about celiac sensitivity, these are gluten-free whole grains, when they're consumed with all of their bran, germ, and endosperm.
** Oats are inherently gluten free but are often contaminated with wheat during growing or processing. There are, however, several brands of pure, uncontaminated oats; ask your doctor if they're acceptable for you.

- **Fill up on beans,** which are a superb source of protein and slowly digested carbs. Try unsalted or low-salt pinto, garbanzo, white, or black beans as a side dish or main protein dish. How easy are they? Open can, heat, and eat.

There's one more terrific secret to healthy weight control, and you'll find it in a beautiful land that resides along the Mediterranean.

The Skinny on Weight Loss Success

The first week I lost about 7 pounds, and by the end of the second week I was down 10 pounds. I was originally at 214 and I got down to about 204.

The diet gave me a broad spectrum of foods to enjoy and to look for in the marketplace. It helped me look at the calories and fat in the foods I choose. Before this, my food mind-set was to reward myself and not pay much attention to what I was eating.

My job involves sitting at my desk a lot; I didn't have enough exercise in my life. You can't lose pounds without a little bit of sacrifice. One thing that Rocco made me aware of was that you don't have to do three hours of exercise a day, but you can do it in several ten-minute spurts, if you get your heart rate up to the right point. Get your metabolism going and you'll burn the fat.

I'm fifty-seven years old, so I had to make a transition to a lower-calorie diet from the more traditional foods I was accustomed to, like burgers and pizza. All in all, the meals on Rocco's plan are satisfying, and the snacks are all good. At times, it felt like I was eating more than I needed to, because I was stopping so often to eat all the snacks.

Rocco really practices what he preaches, and this has challenged me to exercise more and to be self-disciplined and more aware of what I'm eating. It's mind-altering, because it makes you aware of the fact that ultimately it's up to you to be empowered by this kind of weight loss program.

—Roger

CHAPTER 4

Mediterranean Diet Rules Apply

THE MEDIA is on a constant chase to find the perfect diet.

Diet studies are published, the results are often oversimplified and misunderstood, and reporters and dieters stampede in different directions every three months or so.

It reminds me of the old saying about Hollywood, "Nobody knows anything." Sometimes I think the diet world is like that, too.

But there is good news, and it's what this book is based on: Losing weight doesn't have to mean giving up flavor and satisfaction. There are Diet Booster Foods that can help you lose weight. And there is a pattern of healthy eating that is being increasingly championed by the best experts as optimal for both a healthy weight and overall health, a pattern I call a *calorie-corrected*, *carb-corrected*, *Mediterranean-style diet pattern*, a diet pattern that can include versions of almost all of your favorite foods.

As the experts at the Harvard School of Public Health point out, "If you are serious about losing weight, find a diet that appeals to your taste buds." They add, "It should provide plenty of choices, have few restrictions, and be as good for your heart, bones, and brain as it is for your waistline. It should be a diet you are excited about trying, or at least not dreading. Most important, it should deliver fewer calories than you usually take in."

Dr. Walter Willett, the Harvard School of Public Health's healthy-eating guru, nails it for me when he puts it this way in an article titled "Ask the

Expert: Controlling Your Weight" published on the school's website: "The real issue is not losing weight—people can cut back on calories and lose weight on almost any diet—but keeping weight off over the long run. Thus it is more important to find a way of eating that you can stay with for the rest of your life. For this reason, any eating plan you choose should be satisfying and allow variety, and should also be nutritionally sound." And the Mediterranean diet delivers on this, big-time.

The Mediterranean diet is the gold standard of diet patterns, and it's the foundation of the eating plan in **The Pound a Day Diet**. Many of the dishes and recipes in this book are directly inspired or influenced by it, with my new twists and tweaks. And it can totally transform your body and your life.

According to research findings published in the world's leading medical and health journals, the Mediterranean dietary pattern can:

- Lengthen your life

- Improve brain function

- Defend you from chronic diseases

- Fight certain cancers

- Lower your risk of heart disease, high blood pressure, and elevated bad cholesterol levels

- Protect you from type 2 diabetes

- Aid your weight loss and management efforts

- Keep away depression

- Safeguard you from Alzheimer's disease

- Ward off Parkinson's disease

- Ease rheumatoid arthritis

- Improve eye health

- Reduce risk of dental disease

- Help you breathe better

- Lead to healthier babies

- Lead to improved fertility

Best of all, a Mediterranean-style diet can help you **lose weight and keep it off**. A number of studies have shown it to be associated with healthier weight and lower levels of obesity, to be protective against weight gain, and to be an effective pattern for weight loss.

One of the most fascinating studies of the Mediterranean diet conducted with overweight people was performed at the Harvard-affiliated Brigham and Women's Hospital. The study compared weight loss on a moderate-fat Mediterranean diet with weight loss on a low-fat diet in a head-to-head showdown. The Mediterranean diet was high in fruits and vegetables, nuts, and whole grains, with olive oil being the main source of dietary fat. Both test diets stressed controlling portion sizes as a way of reducing calories.

The result? For sustained weight loss over the long haul, the Mediterranean diet rocked. Again, according to Dr. Walter Willett of the Harvard School of Public Health, "The group assigned to the Mediterranean diet lost an average of nine pounds in eighteen months, whereas volunteers assigned to a low-fat diet gained an average of six pounds during that time period. At the study's end, only twenty percent of volunteers in the low-fat group were still following the diet, compared to fifty-four percent of those in the Mediterranean group."

What accounted for the difference in weight loss? The secret boiled down to two words: **pleasure** and **taste**! According to Dr. Willett, "The Mediterranean group volunteers said that their diet regimen was enjoyable and was more flavorful than a low-fat diet."

Pretty simple, right? When you love the way things taste, you're likely to want to eat them over the long term. Other reasons the Mediterranean diet may be so good for your waistline: It's relatively high in low-calorie Diet Booster Foods, it's high in fiber, and it has a low glycemic index.

WHAT EXACTLY IS THE MEDITERRANEAN DIET?

There is no one official definition, but in a nutshell, the Mediterranean diet means high consumption of olive oil, fruits and vegetables (including legumes like beans, peas, and lentils), and unrefined cereals like whole grains; moderate consumption of dairy products, mostly as cheese and yogurt; moderate consumption of wine; moderate-to-high consumption of fish; and low consumption of meat and meat products—all combined with daily physical activity. Meat is enjoyed, but less often than in the US and frequently as more of a garnish than a big main dish. Specifically, here are some major characteristics of the Mediterranean diet pattern, according to the food think tank Oldways Preservation Trust:

- Four or more servings of vegetables a day. A serving is ½ cup of raw or cooked vegetables, 1 cup of raw leafy greens, or ½ cup of vegetable juice.

- Four or more servings of fruit a day. A serving is ½ cup of fresh, frozen, or canned fruit, ¼ cup of dried fruit, one medium-sized piece of fruit, or ½ cup of fruit juice.

- Six or more servings of grain—mostly whole grain—a day. A serving is 1 cup of dry breakfast cereal; ½ cup of cooked cereal, rice, or pasta; or one slice of bread.

- Two or more servings of fish a week. A serving is 4 ounces.

- One serving of yogurt (1 cup) or cheese (1.5 to 2 ounces) a day.

- One serving of beans or nuts a day. For cooked beans, ½ cup is a serving; for nuts, it's a handful (about 1½ ounces).

- If you enjoy alcohol, limit yourself to one or two drinks a day. One drink is 5 ounces of wine, 12 ounces of beer, or 1½ ounces of liquor.

- Olives and olive oil: Olives and olive oil are central to the Mediterranean diet. Olives are universally eaten whole and are widely used for cooking and flavoring in the countries that border the Mediterranean Sea. Olive oil is the principal source of dietary fat used for cooking, for baking, and for dressing salads and vegetables. Extra virgin olive oil is highest in health-promoting fats, phytonutrients, and other important micronutrients.

• Herbs and spices: Herbs and spices add flavors and aromas to foods, reducing the need to add salt or fat when cooking. They are also rich in a broad range of health-promoting antioxidants, and are used liberally in Mediterranean cuisines. Herbs and spices also contribute to the national identities of the various Mediterranean cuisines.

Do You Eat Like a Mediterranean?

Award yourself one point for each Yes. If you score 6 or higher, you're already eating a traditional Mediterranean-style dietary pattern. Congratulations!

	YES	NO
Vegetables (other than potatoes), 4 or more servings a day		
Fruits, 4 or more servings a day		
Whole grains, 2 or more servings a day		
Beans (legumes), 2 or more servings a week		
Nuts, 2 or more servings a week		
Fish, 2 or more servings a week		
Red and processed meat, 1 or fewer servings a day		
Dairy foods, 1 or fewer servings a day		
More unsaturated fat (olive oil and other liquid vegetable oils) than saturated fat (butter, palm oil, bacon fat, etc.)		

Sources: Oldways Preservation Trust, National Institutes of Health, AARP

Now that we've unlocked the secrets of calorie correction, calorie deficits, carb correction, Diet Booster Foods, and the Mediterranean diet—let's put them all to work for you, and blast off the weight!

PART TWO

PHASE 1
ROCCO'S
POUND
A DAY
DIET

CHAPTER 5

Just Days to a New You!

I LIKE results, and I like them fast.

How about you?

For a long time, the prevailing wisdom among many experts has been that slow, gradual weight loss is best—a pound or two or three per week has been the rule of thumb. For many people, that may be quite healthy, effective, and sustainable. But unfortunately, this piece of advice hasn't helped us, as a nation, lose much weight overall.

In fact, it's getting worse: *USA Today* recently reported that the Centers for Disease Control and Prevention estimates the national obesity rate at 36 percent, and some experts predict that a staggering 42 to 50 percent of Americans will be obese by 2030. Obesity-related illnesses are already costing the US from $147 billion to $210 billion a year.

From experience, I've come to realize that one of the reasons many diets don't work is because they just don't deliver results fast enough—the dieter gets bored and falls off the diet. They're not inspired or motivated; they're frustrated and impatient. At the same time, there are excellent scientific and medical arguments against most fad diets and crash diets that promise fast weight loss. They usually don't work, either, and can pose health risks. Crash diets, extended fasts, medically unsupervised "cleanses," and starvation diets can give you fast weight loss, but who can keep that up for more than a few days at most? Plus, who would want to? Why suffer?

In most cases of people who have enjoyed effective, lasting weight loss (other than via surgery), one of the keys has been reducing the average calorie intake over time, and often also improving the calorie balance with physical activity.

To this end, doctors and scientists have long supported the use of lower-calorie diets, across a wide spectrum of diet patterns. Historically, liquid diet replacement meals have often been used for much-lower-calorie diets under medical supervision, especially for obese patients. The research on the long-term effectiveness of partial or full liquid diets is mixed, but one thing most experts agree on is the critical need to correct your calorie balance by reducing it, if you want to lose weight and keep it off.

The Pound a Day Diet is a low-calorie diet and healthy eating plan. Phase 1, my twenty-eight-day plan, was developed with the guidance of a medical doctor who is also a weight loss expert, as well as a registered dietitian, and it's based on some of the latest research and scientific insights on healthy weight loss.

You'll eat 850 calories per day for five days, and increase to 1,200 calories a day on my weekend plan. And with my detailed meal plans, I predict you'll be satisfied and happy with the food you're enjoying, even if it's significantly less calories than you're currently eating. Now, 850 calories a day is an ambitious, aggressive target, and it is a low-calorie diet, or as I prefer to think of my approach, a healthy eating plan. So, as I've said earlier, you should check with your doctor before beginning this or any other diet.

What does the research say about how safe and effective low-calorie diets are?

In 2006, the *Canadian Medical Association Journal* published a research review on low-calorie diets titled "Diet in the Management of Weight Loss." The authors concluded that "low-calorie diets can lower total body weight by an average of 8 percent in the short term. These diets are well-tolerated and characterize successful strategies in maintaining significant weight loss over a five-year period. Very-low-calorie diets [often defined as 800 calories or less] produce a more rapid weight loss but should only be used for fewer than sixteen weeks because of clinical adverse effects."

The researchers reported that "low-calorie diets should be high in fiber and have a low glycemic index," which is the formula you'll follow in *The Pound a Day Diet*. They also reported on earlier research based on the "gold standard" of randomized controlled trials, which found that "low-calorie diets can lower total body weight by an average of about 8 percent during a period of three to twelve months," and "low-calorie diets resulting in weight loss also lower the amount of abdominal fat, as shown by a reduction in waist circumference of 1.5 to 9.5 cm." They concluded, "Overall, low-calorie diets are a safe strategy for weight loss," and they suggested a sample 1,200-calorie-a-day diet based on a healthy, sustainable eating pattern.

Talk with Your Doctor or Health Professional

Although the definitions can vary, a moderately restricted-calorie diet or low-calorie diet, or LCD, is often considered to be 850 to 1,200 calories per day. A very-low-calorie diet, or VLCD, is often considered to be less than 800 calories a day and usually relies heavily on liquid meal replacements; and an extremely low-calorie diet, or ELCD, can be as low as 500 calories a day and be all liquid. Neither a VLCD nor an ELCD should ever be attempted without a medical doctor's direct supervision, as the lower in calories you go, the higher the health risks, like gallstones, gout, electrolyte disorders, and cardiac and other complications.

But I believe it's a good idea for you to consult with a doctor before attempting any weight loss regimen, including this one. The calorie targets in this diet are ambitious and should be adjusted if necessary by you and your doctor, according to your individual health profile. If you're a man on the larger side, for example, your doctor may want to increase the number of calories you consume during Phase 1, which you can easily do by having extra portions based on the calorie counts on pages 54–64.

I suggest you and your doctor update all your current health stats and establish a baseline to track your progress in the days and weeks ahead.

If you can, you should also hook up with a registered dietitian nutritionist before starting this or any other weight loss plan. I've been working with RDNs for years. An RDN can be your superstar coach for healthy weight loss and healthy eating. In the United States, anyone can call himself or herself a nutritionist. But to be a registered dietitian you've got to go through a rigorous professional credential program. RDNs know more about nutrition and healthy weight loss than a lot of doctors. Look for the credential RDN. That way, you know if someone calling himself or herself a nutritionist or a dietary counselor is among the best qualified.

RDNs work for hospitals, for schools, and in private practice, and several supermarket chains are hiring RDNs you can consult with right in the store. This is brilliant! See if your insurance company or employer will cover the cost of a consultation with an RDN.

I based the plan on the latest research on health, nutrition, and weight loss, including the principles of using a low-calorie diet to create a calorie deficit; using low-calorie-density foods, or Diet Booster Foods, to enhance weight loss; and transitioning to a Mediterranean dietary and lifestyle pattern to stay at a healthy weight over the long term.

The plan assumes that like many adult Americans you are overweight or obese, for example, twenty or thirty pounds over a normal weight; you're probably consuming as much as 4,000 calories or more per day, when you should be consuming roughly half that amount to maintain a healthy weight. The typical unhealthy American diet also features too much sodium and saturated fat and refined sugars—and not enough good fat, good carbs, and fruits and vegetables. **The Pound a Day Diet** also assumes that—again like most Americans—you're relatively sedentary and are not getting recommended levels of average daily physical activity.

Phase 1 is a twenty-eight-day plan of super-delicious, healthy meals and recipes (including ready-made substitutions if you don't have time to cook) totaling between 850 and 1,200 calories a day. It's based on the scientifically validated method of creating a calorie deficit that triggers weight loss; and in this case, using a calorie deficit to trigger steady weight loss over a twenty-eight-day period. Phase 1 is also based on the rule of thumb widely used among experts that a 3,500-calorie deficit results in a pound of weight loss. This is only a rough guideline, and your weight loss can vary depending on your starting weight, sex, body type, motivation, and other factors. During Phase 1 you may lose anywhere from a few pounds a week to five pounds or more. Over the course of twenty-eight days, you can lose up to twenty pounds!

Remember why you're doing this: You care about yourself, your health, and your friends and family. Today is the day you decided to get really serious about getting healthy. Stick with it and just wait till you see the pounds fly off and how good it feels when you get into your skinny jeans and you start to feel better and better. It's pure bliss!

Now let's get you started on your journey to fast, healthy weight loss!

THE COMPLETE PHASE 1 WEIGHT LOSS PLAN

Phase 1 incorporates the weight loss principles outlined in Part 1. It's a calorie-corrected, carb-corrected healthy eating program that uses specific meal plans.

The recipes were designed by me and were created using my twenty-five years of experience as a chef, as well as my knowledge of healthy eating and flavor. This turbocharged weight loss plan is:

- *Calorie corrected*, which means it's designed to give you a calorie deficit for steady, fast weight loss results, and to bring you toward calorie balance for the long term. You'll eat 850 calories a day for five days a week, and then increase to 1,200 calories a day for two days a week.

- *Carb corrected*, which means you'll be cutting out most refined carbohydrates from your diet and getting most of your carbs from vegetable sources.

- *Based on Diet Booster Foods* that are low in calorie density, to help you lose weight and feel fuller sooner and to protect you from over-eating. These include lots of fruits and veggies, among other delicious foods.

- *Nutritionally balanced,* so you include a healthy mix of nutrients in your diet. This healthy balance will keep you from feeling hungry and will give you the energy you need. It's also high in protein, which many studies have suggested is an effective pathway to weight loss.

- *Designed with the idea that you will take charge and cook for yourself,* but it also has store-bought solutions for when you're in a hurry. When you cook for yourself, you know exactly what's in your meal and you can better keep track of your calorie consumption.

Specifically, here's how the plan works: Every weekday, you'll eat three meals and two snacks that add up to 850 calories. Then on the weekends, you'll eat three meals and two snacks that add up to 1,200 calories per day. You'll follow specially formulated meal plans I've designed, for up to twenty-eight days—less if you reach your goal weight sooner.

Phase 1

Exercise Recommendation: Start Power-Walking—at Least Thirty Minutes a Day

To help maximize your calorie deficit, improve your overall fitness and health, and boost your potential weight loss in Phase 1, I recommend that on almost every day of the twenty-eight days you do a moderate-intensity exercise like power-walking at a brisk pace.

You can break it down to three bursts of at least ten minutes spread throughout the day if you like.

Practically anybody can begin a power-walking program. The only special equipment you need is a decent pair of sneakers, and all you need to do is get out and walk!

It's the easiest exercise in the world! And it works. If you weigh 163 pounds and you power-walk for just thirty-three minutes at a very brisk pace of four miles an hour, for example, you'll burn off 203 calories, according to myfitnesspal.com. More details on exercise and physical activity are given in chapter 8.

I've provided four five-day plans, plus four weekend meal plans—all organized into a twenty-eight-day eating program. Day by day, you may witness a remarkable transformation in yourself—and see the evidence on your scale and in your mirror, as pounds and inches steadily disappear.

If you're committed to a slimmer you—and I hope you are—get ready to knock off pounds right away! For every day that you stick to the diet plan, you can expect to lose up to a pound a day, depending on your personal health profile and your commitment. Start following this simple plan now, and watch the flab melt away.

Weigh yourself once a week and record your weight loss. You don't need to weigh yourself every day. Scales are a good benchmark on your progress, but they're also an obsession that can take over your life.

As soon as you reach your target weight, which could be the healthy body mass index weight detailed on pages 223-224, stop Phase 1 and go right to Phase 2, the Maintenance Phase, which is chapter 7, beginning on page 221.

PHASE 1: OVERVIEW

HOW TO BEGIN

- Follow the twenty-eight-day meal plans.
- Before beginning the diet, review your health stats, and the diet, with your doctor.
- If you reach your goal weight before the twenty-eight days are over, stop Phase 1 and go straight to Phase 2, the Maintenance Phase.

AVERAGE CALORIE OVERVIEW

Day 1:	850 calories
Day 2:	850 calories
Day 3:	850 calories
Day 4:	850 calories
Day 5:	850 calories
Day 6:	1,200 calories
Day 7:	1,200 calories—*weigh yourself*
Day 8:	850 calories
Day 9:	850 calories
Day 10:	850 calories

Day 11:   850 calories

Day 12:   850 calories

Day 13:   1,200 calories

Day 14:   1,200 calories—*weigh yourself*

Day 15:   850 calories

Day 16:   850 calories

Day 17:   850 calories

Day 18:   850 calories

Day 19:   850 calories

Day 20:   1,200 calories

Day 21:   1,200 calories—*weigh yourself*

Day 22:   850 calories

Day 23:   850 calories

Day 24:   850 calories

Day 25:   850 calories

Day 26:   850 calories

Day 27:   1,200 calories

Day 28:   1,200 calories—*weigh yourself*

MEAL PLANS AND SHOPPING LISTS FOR FAST RESULTS

I'm including meal plans for all twenty-eight days and shopping lists to help you get started. Many of the suggested meals and snacks have corresponding recipes that you can find in the next chapter. All the recipes are simple and delicious. And if you don't have time to cook, I've suggested ready-made substitutions that you'll find helpful.

It's extremely important that you do not skip meals. That's called fasting. When you fast, your body stores energy as fat, and that causes weight gain, not weight loss.

Eat every two and a half to three hours. Even if you're not hungry, eat a little bit of what's in the meal plan to keep your metabolic system revving high all day.

Please drink plenty of water! Water is necessary to flush toxins, detox from all the processed foods, keep you feeling full, and keep your metabolism firing on all cylinders. The plan assumes that water is usually your main beverage with meals, except when otherwise noted. Nonfat milk is fine, too, as are unsweetened coffee, black tea, green tea, and herbal tea.

Do not drink soda of any kind. Even diet sodas are not OK. The only drinks allowed are water and real brewed tea, either iced or hot, sweetened with monk fruit or stevia.

I believe that taking a multivitamin for nutritional insurance is a good idea. Consult with your doctor about taking a multivitamin or other supplements, and about all aspects of this plan as it applies to your personal health profile, and any necessary revisions. The calorie counts below refer to the recipes and calories-per-serving that are listed in chapter 6. Calories are rounded to the nearest calorie; the key source for calorie information is calorieking.com.

THE POUND A DAY DIET MEAL PLANS
Phase 1

DAY 1

		CALORIES
BREAKFAST	High-Protein Chocolate Breakfast Smoothie	198
	Grapefruit with Zero-Calorie Spiced "Sugar"	28
SNACK 1	Super Popcorn-Kale Crumble	40
LUNCH	Salmon and Cucumber Salad with Creamy Dill Dressing	171
SNACK 2	The Green Monkey	77
DINNER	Beef and Broccoli Stir-Fry	193
DINNER SIDE	1 cup iceberg lettuce, 5 cherry tomatoes, 1 teaspoon red wine vinegar	29
BEVERAGE	Green Tea with Lemon and Basil	4
DESSERT	Fresh Raspberries with Sugar-Free Vanilla Cream	83
TOTAL CALORIES		823

DAY 2

		CALORIES
BREAKFAST	High-Protein Chocolate Breakfast Smoothie	198
	Grapefruit with Zero-Calorie Spiced "Sugar"	28
SNACK 1	All-Day Egg-White Omelet with Pico de Gallo	70
LUNCH	Rotisserie Chicken and Teriyaki Asian Noodles	187
SNACK 2	Almond Milk Smoothie	84
DINNER	Salmon Teriyaki with Grapefruit and Fennel	210
BEVERAGE	Southern-Style Sweet Tea	3
DESSERT	Fresh Strawberries with Sugar-Free Chocolate Sauce	49
TOTAL CALORIES		829

DAY 3

		CALORIES
BREAKFAST	High-Protein Chocolate Breakfast Smoothie	198
	Grapefruit with Zero-Calorie Spiced "Sugar"	28
SNACK 1	1 cup broccoli with 2 tablespoons hummus	72
LUNCH	Old-Fashioned Chicken Noodle Soup	191

		CALORIES
SNACK 2	Fresh Wasabi Peas	29
DINNER	Bacon-Wrapped Chicken with Sweet Rutabaga Mash	232
BEVERAGE	Green Tea with Lemon and Basil	4
DESSERT	High-Protein "Rice" Pudding with Papaya	81
TOTAL CALORIES		835

DAY 4

		CALORIES
BREAKFAST	High-Protein Chocolate Breakfast Smoothie	198
	Grapefruit with Zero-Calorie Spiced "Sugar"	28
SNACK 1	Apples and Cheddar Cheese	117
LUNCH	Grilled Shrimp Gazpacho	140
SNACK 2	The Green Monkey	77
DINNER	Thai Noodles with Turkey	199
BEVERAGE	Southern-Style Sweet Tea	3
DESSERT	Frozen Dark Chocolate Shake	91
TOTAL CALORIES		853

DAY 5

		CALORIES
BREAKFAST	High-Protein Chocolate Breakfast Smoothie	198
	Grapefruit with Zero-Calorie Spiced "Sugar"	28
SNACK 1	Sweet Potato Chips	37
LUNCH	Turkey and Lentil Soup	204
SNACK 2	Almond Milk Smoothie	84
DINNER	Salisbury Steak with Mushroom Gravy	178
DINNER SIDE	1 cup iceberg lettuce, 5 cherry tomatoes, 1 teaspoon red wine vinegar	29
BEVERAGE	Green Tea with Lemon and Basil	4
DESSERT	Fresh Raspberries with Sugar-Free Vanilla Cream	83
TOTAL CALORIES		845

DAY 6

		CALORIES
BREAKFAST	High-Protein Chocolate Breakfast Smoothie	198
	Grapefruit with Zero-Calorie Spiced "Sugar"	28
	Protein-Packed Breakfast Sandwich	188
SNACK 1	Super Popcorn-Kale Crumble	40
	Almonds, 6	42
LUNCH	BBQ Chicken Cutlets	129
	1 cup cherry tomatoes	27
SNACK 2	The Green Monkey	77
DINNER	Chicken Enchiladas	225
	½ avocado	161
DESSERT	Instant Vanilla Frozen Yogurt in a Blender	86
TOTAL CALORIES		1,201

DAY 7

		CALORIES
BREAKFAST	High-Protein Chocolate Breakfast Smoothie	198
	Protein-Packed Breakfast Sandwich	188
SNACK 1	Grapefruit with Zero-Calorie Spiced "Sugar"	28
LUNCH	Mediterranean Tuna Salad	90
SNACK 2	Apples and Cheddar Cheese	117
DINNER	Turkey Alfredo	206
DINNER SIDE	1 cup iceberg lettuce, 5 cherry tomatoes, 1 teaspoon red wine vinegar	29
	½ avocado	161
DESSERT	Instant Chocolate Soft-Serve in a Juicer	82
TOTAL CALORIES		1099

DAY 8

		CALORIES
BREAKFAST	High-Protein Chocolate Breakfast Smoothie	198
	Grapefruit with Zero-Calorie Spiced "Sugar"	28
SNACK 1	1 cup broccoli with 2 tablespoons hummus	72
LUNCH	Crunchy Kale, Apple, and Pomegranate Salad	126
	3 ounces boneless, skinless store-roasted turkey breast	115

		CALORIES
SNACK 2	Banana Cream Smoothie	103
DINNER	Roasted Turkey with Green Beans and Gravy	138
BEVERAGE	Green Tea with Lemon and Basil	4
DESSERT	High-Protein "Rice" Pudding with Papaya	81
TOTAL CALORIES		865

DAY 9

		CALORIES
BREAKFAST	High-Protein Chocolate Breakfast Smoothie	198
	Grapefruit with Zero-Calorie Spiced "Sugar"	28
SNACK 1	All-Day Egg-White Omelet with Pico de Gallo	70
LUNCH	Tomato and Shrimp Kimchi Salad	116
SNACK 2	The Green Monkey	77
DINNER	Bacon-Wrapped Chicken with Sweet Rutabaga Mash	232
DINNER SIDE	1 cup iceberg lettuce, 5 cherry tomatoes, 1 teaspoon red wine vinegar	29
BEVERAGE	Southern-Style Sweet Tea	3
DESSERT	Frozen Strawberry Shake	81
TOTAL CALORIES		834

DAY 10

		CALORIES
BREAKFAST	High-Protein Chocolate Breakfast Smoothie	198
	Grapefruit with Zero-Calorie Spiced "Sugar"	28
SNACK 1	Greek Yogurt with Crunchy Blueberry Topping	142
LUNCH	Salmon and Cucumber Salad with Creamy Dill Dressing	171
SNACK 2	Almond Milk Smoothie	84
DINNER	Sweet Sesame Turkey with Bok Choy	147
BEVERAGE	Green Tea with Lemon and Basil	4
DESSERT	High-Protein "Rice" Pudding with Papaya	81
TOTAL CALORIES		855

DAY 11

		CALORIES
BREAKFAST	High-Protein Chocolate Breakfast Smoothie	198
	Grapefruit with Zero-Calorie Spiced "Sugar"	28
SNACK 1	Apples and Cheddar Cheese	117
	Almonds, 8	55
LUNCH	Lemon Garlic Shrimp Pasta	105
SNACK 2	The Green Monkey	77
DINNER	Salisbury Steak with Mushroom Gravy	178
BEVERAGE	Southern-Style Sweet Tea	3
DESSERT	Frozen Dark Chocolate Shake	91
TOTAL CALORIES		852

DAY 12

		CALORIES
BREAKFAST	High-Protein Chocolate Breakfast Smoothie	198
	Grapefruit with Zero-Calorie Spiced "Sugar"	28
SNACK 1	Sweet Potato Chips	37
LUNCH	Old-Fashioned Chicken Noodle Soup	191
SNACK 2	Fresh Wasabi Peas	29
	Almonds, 10	69
DINNER	Pork Cutlet alla Pizzaiola	193
DINNER SIDE	1 cup iceberg lettuce, 5 cherry tomatoes, 1 teaspoon red wine vinegar	29
BEVERAGE	Green Tea with Lemon and Basil	4
DESSERT	Fresh Raspberries with Sugar-Free Vanilla Cream	83
TOTAL CALORIES		861

DAY 13

		CALORIES
BREAKFAST	High-Protein Chocolate Breakfast Smoothie	198
	Protein-Packed Breakfast Sandwich	188
	Grapefruit with Zero-Calorie Spiced "Sugar"	28
SNACK 1	All-Day Egg-White Omelet with Pico de Gallo	70
LUNCH	BBQ Chicken Cutlets	129
	Virgin Mary	46

		CALORIES
SNACK 2	The Green Monkey	77
DINNER	Salmon Teriyaki with Grapefruit and Fennel	210
	½ avocado	161
DESSERT	Instant Vanilla Frozen Yogurt in a Blender	86
TOTAL CALORIES		1193

DAY 14

		CALORIES
BREAKFAST	High-Protein Chocolate Breakfast Smoothie	198
	Protein-Packed Breakfast Sandwich	188
	Grapefruit with Zero-Calorie Spiced "Sugar"	28
SNACK 1	Greek Yogurt with Crunchy Blueberry Topping	142
LUNCH	Mediterranean Tuna Salad	90
SNACK 2	Almond Milk Smoothie	84
DINNER	Beef and Broccoli Stir-Fry	193
	2 tablespoons pickled ginger	40
	½ avocado	161
DESSERT	Instant Chocolate Soft-Serve in a Juicer	82
TOTAL CALORIES		1,206

DAY 15

		CALORIES
BREAKFAST	High-Protein Chocolate Breakfast Smoothie	198
	Grapefruit with Zero-Calorie Spiced "Sugar"	28
SNACK 1	Super Popcorn-Kale Crumble	40
LUNCH	Rotisserie Chicken and Teriyaki Asian Noodles	187
SNACK 2	The Green Monkey	77
DINNER	Thai Noodles with Turkey	199
BEVERAGE	Green Tea with Lemon and Basil	4
DESSERT	Frozen Strawberry Shake	81
TOTAL CALORIES		814

DAY 16

		CALORIES
BREAKFAST	High-Protein Chocolate Breakfast Smoothie	198
	Grapefruit with Zero-Calorie Spiced "Sugar"	28
SNACK 1	All-Day Egg-White Omelet with Pico de Gallo	70
LUNCH	BBQ Chicken Cutlets	129
	1 ounce 75% reduced-fat cheddar	60
SNACK 2	Almond Milk Smoothie	84
DINNER	Chicken Enchiladas	225
BEVERAGE	Southern-Style Sweet Tea	3
DESSERT	Fresh Strawberries with Sugar-Free Chocolate Sauce	49
TOTAL CALORIES		846

DAY 17

		CALORIES
BREAKFAST	High-Protein Chocolate Breakfast Smoothie	198
	Grapefruit with Zero-Calorie Spiced "Sugar"	28
SNACK 1	Greek Yogurt with Crunchy Blueberry Topping	142
LUNCH	Lemon Garlic Shrimp Pasta	105
	1 cup cherry tomatoes	27
SNACK 2	Fresh Wasabi Peas	29
DINNER	Bacon-Wrapped Chicken with Sweet Rutabaga Mash	232
BEVERAGE	Green Tea with Lemon and Basil	4
DESSERT	Fresh Raspberries with Sugar-Free Vanilla Cream	83
TOTAL CALORIES		848

DAY 18

		CALORIES
BREAKFAST	High-Protein Chocolate Breakfast Smoothie	198
	Grapefruit with Zero-Calorie Spiced "Sugar"	28
SNACK 1	Apples and Cheddar Cheese	117
LUNCH	Grilled Shrimp Gazpacho	140
	1/4 avocado	80
SNACK 2	The Green Monkey	77
DINNER	Sweet Sesame Turkey with Bok Choy	147
BEVERAGE	Southern-Style Sweet Tea	3
DESSERT	Frozen Strawberry Shake	81
TOTAL CALORIES		871

DAY 19

		CALORIES
BREAKFAST	High-Protein Chocolate Breakfast Smoothie	198
	Grapefruit with Zero-Calorie Spiced "Sugar"	28
SNACK 1	Sweet Potato Chips	37
LUNCH	Salmon and Cucumber Salad with Creamy Dill Dressing	171
SNACK 2	Banana Cream Smoothie	103
DINNER	Turkey Alfredo	206
DINNER SIDE	1 cup iceberg lettuce, 5 cherry tomatoes, 1 teaspoon red wine vinegar	29
BEVERAGE	Green Tea with Lemon and Basil	4
DESSERT	Rocco's Quick-Fill Chocolate-Strawberry Bar	82
TOTAL CALORIES		858

DAY 20

		CALORIES
BREAKFAST	High-Protein Chocolate Breakfast Smoothie	198
	Grapefruit with Zero-Calorie Spiced "Sugar"	28
	Protein-Packed Breakfast Sandwich	188
SNACK 1	Greek Yogurt with Crunchy Blueberry Topping	142
LUNCH	Manhattan Clam Chowder	122
SNACK 2	1 cup broccoli with 2 tablespoons hummus	72
DINNER	Beef and Broccoli Stir-Fry	193
	½ avocado	161
DESSERT	Instant Vanilla Frozen Yogurt in a Blender	86
TOTAL CALORIES		1,190

DAY 21

		CALORIES
BREAKFAST	High-Protein Chocolate Breakfast Smoothie	198
	Grapefruit with Zero-Calorie Spiced "Sugar"	28
	Protein-Packed Breakfast Sandwich	188
SNACK 1	All-Day Egg-White Omelet with Pico de Gallo	70
LUNCH	Southwestern Rice and Bean Salad with Cheddar Cheese	182
SNACK 2	Almond Milk Smoothie	84

(continued)

		CALORIES
DINNER	Salmon Teriyaki with Grapefruit and Fennel	**210**
	½ avocado	**161**
DESSERT	Instant Chocolate Soft-Serve in a Juicer	**82**
TOTAL CALORIES		**1,203**

DAY 22

		CALORIES
BREAKFAST	High-Protein Chocolate Breakfast Smoothie	**198**
	Grapefruit with Zero-Calorie Spiced "Sugar"	**28**
SNACK 1	Super Popcorn-Kale Crumble	**40**
LUNCH	Salmon and Cucumber Salad with Creamy Dill Dressing	**171**
SNACK 2	The Green Monkey	**77**
DINNER	Bacon-Wrapped Chicken with Sweet Rutabaga Mash	**232**
BEVERAGE	Green Tea with Lemon and Basil	**4**
DESSERT	Fresh Raspberries with Sugar-Free Vanilla Cream	**83**
TOTAL CALORIES		**833**

DAY 23

		CALORIES
BREAKFAST	High-Protein Chocolate Breakfast Smoothie	**198**
	Grapefruit with Zero-Calorie Spiced "Sugar"	**28**
SNACK 1	Apples and Cheddar Cheese	**117**
LUNCH	Crunchy Kale, Apple, and Pomegranate Salad	**126**
	3 ounces boneless, skinless store-roasted turkey breast	**115**
SNACK 2	Fresh Wasabi Peas	**29**
DINNER	Thai Noodles with Turkey	**199**
BEVERAGE	Southern-Style Sweet Tea	**3**
DESSERT	Fresh Strawberries with Sugar-Free Chocolate Sauce	**49**
TOTAL CALORIES		**864**

DAY 24

		CALORIES
BREAKFAST	High-Protein Chocolate Breakfast Smoothie	198
	Grapefruit with Zero-Calorie Spiced "Sugar"	28
SNACK 1	Greek Yogurt with Crunchy Blueberry Topping	142
LUNCH	Rotisserie Chicken and Teriyaki Asian Noodles	187
SNACK 2	Almond Milk Smoothie	84
DINNER	Roasted Turkey with Green Beans and Gravy	138
BEVERAGE	Green Tea with Lemon and Basil	4
DESSERT	High-Protein "Rice" Pudding with Papaya	81
TOTAL CALORIES		862

DAY 25

		CALORIES
BREAKFAST	High-Protein Chocolate Breakfast Smoothie	198
	Grapefruit with Zero-Calorie Spiced "Sugar"	28
SNACK 1	Super Popcorn-Kale Crumble	40
LUNCH	Grilled Shrimp Gazpacho	140
	1 ounce 75% reduced-fat cheddar	60
SNACK 2	1 cup broccoli with 2 tablespoons hummus	72
DINNER	Pork Cutlet alla Pizzaiola	193
DINNER SIDE	1 cup iceberg lettuce, 5 cherry tomatoes, 1 teaspoon red wine vinegar	29
BEVERAGE	Southern-Style Sweet Tea	3
DESSERT	Frozen Dark Chocolate Shake	91
TOTAL CALORIES		854

DAY 26

		CALORIES
BREAKFAST	High-Protein Chocolate Breakfast Smoothie	198
	Grapefruit with Zero-Calorie Spiced "Sugar"	28
SNACK 1	Sweet Potato Chips	37
LUNCH	Turkey and Lentil Soup	204
SNACK 2	The Green Monkey	77
DINNER	Salisbury Steak with Mushroom Gravy	178

(continued)

		CALORIES
DINNER SIDE	1 cup iceberg lettuce, 5 cherry tomatoes, 1 teaspoon red wine vinegar	29
BEVERAGE	Green Tea with Lemon and Basil	4
DESSERT	Fresh Raspberries with Sugar-Free Vanilla Cream	83
TOTAL CALORIES		838

DAY 27

		CALORIES
BREAKFAST	High-Protein Chocolate Breakfast Smoothie	198
	Grapefruit with Zero-Calorie Spiced "Sugar"	28
	Protein-Packed Breakfast Sandwich	188
SNACK 1	All-Day Egg-White Omelet with Pico de Gallo	70
LUNCH	Mediterranean Tuna Salad	90
SNACK 2	Banana Cream Smoothie	103
DINNER	Chicken Enchiladas	225
DINNER SIDE	1 cup iceberg lettuce, 5 cherry tomatoes, 1 teaspoon red wine vinegar	29
	½ avocado	161
BEVERAGE	Southern-Style Sweet Tea	3
DESSERT	Instant Vanilla Frozen Yogurt in a Blender	86
TOTAL CALORIES		1,181

DAY 28

		CALORIES
BREAKFAST	High-Protein Chocolate Breakfast Smoothie	198
	Grapefruit with Zero-Calorie Spiced "Sugar"	28
	Protein-Packed Breakfast Sandwich	188
SNACK 1	Super Popcorn-Kale Crumble	40
LUNCH	Southwestern Rice and Bean Salad with Cheddar Cheese	182
SNACK 2	The Green Monkey	77
DINNER	Beef and Broccoli Stir-Fry	193
DINNER SIDE	1 cup cherry tomatoes	27
	½ avocado	161
DESSERT	Instant Chocolate Soft-Serve in a Juicer	82
TOTAL CALORIES		1,176

SHOPPING LISTS

Note: These shopping lists are designed for four people.

PHASE 1, WEEK 1

PRODUCE

- [ ] 6 large bunches kale
- [ ] 14 Ruby Red grapefruits
- [ ] 8 lemons
- [ ] 2 bunches dill
- [ ] 2 bunches basil
- [ ] 2 quarts undressed cucumber, red onion, and cherry tomato salad (find in salad bar section or deli counter at supermarket)
- [ ] 4 large cucumbers or 6 small-to-medium cucumbers
- [ ] 6 Granny Smith apples
- [ ] 2 pints chopped carrots (check produce department or salad bar)
- [ ] 2 bags frozen broccoli florets
- [ ] 4 pints cherry tomatoes
- [ ] 2 heads iceberg lettuce
- [ ] 2 pints fresh raspberries
- [ ] 2 small packets freeze-dried raspberries (optional)
- [ ] 2 bunches mint (optional)
- [ ] 4 pints mild pico de gallo (such as Ready Pac)
- [ ] 2 pints spicy pico de gallo (such as Ready Pac)
- [ ] 2 bunches cilantro
- [ ] 2 medium fennel bulbs
- [ ] 2 pints (fresh packed) grapefruit sections
- [ ] 2 pints fresh strawberries
- [ ] 2 pints fresh broccoli florets
- [ ] 2 small containers hummus (look for 50 calories per serving, such as Athenos)
- [ ] 4 pints precut fresh mirepoix (diced onion, carrot, celery—look in produce department)
- [ ] 2 bags cleaned fresh sugar snap peas
- [ ] 2 medium rutabagas
- [ ] 1 papaya or 2 small papayas
- [ ] 8 small apples (such as Pink Lady, Gala, or Winesap)
- [ ] 2 cups store-cut vegetable mix (broccoli, cauliflower, peppers, etc.)
- [ ] 2 bags frozen sliced mixed bell peppers and onions (such as Birds Eye Pepper and Onion Stir-Fry)
- [ ] 2 bags no-sugar-added frozen strawberries
- [ ] 2 sweet potatoes

- ☐ 2 bags (find in produce section) or can ready-to-eat cooked lentils (such as Melissa's or Eden)
- ☐ 2 pints fresh chopped vegetable medley (such as Salad Confetti by Ready Pac)
- ☐ 2 heads butter lettuce
- ☐ 2 underripe bananas
- ☐ 4 avocados

DAIRY, EGGS, BREAD

- ☐ Two 35-ounce containers fat-free Greek yogurt (such as Fage Total 0%)
- ☐ 2 small bottles liquid sugar-free vanilla coffee creamer (such as Coffee-Mate)
- ☐ 6 blocks 75% reduced-fat cheddar cheese (such as Cabot)
- ☐ 1 gallon unsweetened vanilla almond milk (such as Silk)
- ☐ 2 pints nonfat cottage cheese (such as Friendship)
- ☐ 2 pints egg whites
- ☐ 2 small chunks Pecorino Romano
- ☐ 2 pints fat-free milk
- ☐ 2 pints egg replacement (such as Egg Beaters)
- ☐ 2 packages fat-free American cheese (such as Kraft)
- ☐ 2 packages light whole-wheat hamburger buns (such as Sara Lee Delightful Wheat)

PROTEIN

- ☐ Two 8-ounce cans sockeye salmon
- ☐ 12 ounces grass-fed beef tenderloin
- ☐ 3 store-roasted chickens
- ☐ 16 ounces salmon filet (wild sockeye, Chinook, or king is preferable)
- ☐ 8 boneless, skinless chicken breast cutlets (4 ounces each)
- ☐ 2 packs turkey bacon (such as Butterball Everyday Thin & Crispy)
- ☐ 16 ounces store-prepared boiled shrimp, shells removed
- ☐ 24 ounces sliced turkey breast, sliced ¼ inch thick at deli
- ☐ 12 ounces 96% lean ground beef (such as Laura's Lean)
- ☐ 2 boxes turkey breakfast sausage patties (such as Bob Evans)

DRY GOODS/PANTRY

- ☐ 1 canister psyllium husk powder
- ☐ 1 canister fiber powder (such as ReNew Life Triple Fiber)
- ☐ 1 canister protein powder (such as Daily Benefit)
- ☐ 1 pound dark unsweetened cocoa powder (such as Hershey's Special Dark)
- ☐ 10 boxes monk fruit extract (such as Monk Fruit In The Raw, 40-count box)

- ☐ 2 packs plain air-popped popcorn (4 cups each)
- ☐ 4 cans olive oil spray (such as Pam)
- ☐ 1 bottle red wine vinegar
- ☐ 1 canister crushed red pepper flakes
- ☐ 1 canister cayenne pepper
- ☐ 1 canister cinnamon powder
- ☐ 1 canister ginger powder
- ☐ 4 packages instant sugar-free banana cream or vanilla pudding mix (such as Jell-O)
- ☐ 4 packages instant sugar-free vanilla pudding mix (such as Jell-O)
- ☐ 2 package instant brown gravy (such as Knorr)
- ☐ 4 bottles reduced-sodium sugar-free teriyaki sauce (such as Seal Sama)
- ☐ Four 6-ounce bags shirataki rice (such as Miracle Noodle—substitute a different shirataki product and chop it up if the rice cut is unavailable)
- ☐ 4 ounces unsalted almonds
- ☐ 2 boxes black tea (such as Lipton)
- ☐ 2 boxes green tea (such as sencha)
- ☐ 2 bags xanthan gum (such as Bob's Red Mill)
- ☐ Twelve 6-ounce sugar-free reduced-calorie vanilla pudding cups (such as Jell-O)
- ☐ 2 jars pickled cherry peppers
- ☐ 32 ounces tofu shirataki noodles
- ☐ 1 bottle almond extract
- ☐ Two 24-ounce bag unflavored egg-white powder (such as Jay Robb)
- ☐ 1 canister no-added-salt-or-sugar wasabi powder (such as Eden)
- ☐ 1 bottle raw agave nectar
- ☐ 2 bags (8.29 ounces) zero-calorie all-natural sweetener (such as Lakanto)
- ☐ 4 quarts fat-free, unsalted chicken stock or broth (such as Kitchen Basics or Swanson's)
- ☐ 2 small boxes salt-free vegetable bouillon cubes (such as Rapunzel)
- ☐ Six 8-ounce bags shirataki spaghetti
- ☐ 1 jar no-added-sugar-or-salt peanut butter (such as Smucker's Natural)
- ☐ 1 canister red curry paste
- ☐ 2 bags organic fat-free milk powder (such as Organic Valley)
- ☐ 1 canister seafood seasoning (such as Old Bay)
- ☐ 1 canister sweet smoked paprika
- ☐ 2 cans 98% fat-free cream of mushroom soup (such as Campbell's)

- [ ] 2 small boxes or cans (8.25 ounces) unsalted beef stock (such as Kitchen Basics)
- [ ] 16 ounces shirataki macaroni
- [ ] 1 bottle liquid smoke
- [ ] 2 bottles reduced-sugar ketchup (such as Heinz)
- [ ] 1 bottle all-natural or pure vanilla extract
- [ ] 1 bottle brined capers
- [ ] 2 cans water-packed, no-salt-added tuna (such as Sustainable Seas)
- [ ] 16 original, small-size, low-carb tortillas (such as La Tortilla Factory)
- [ ] 2 canisters vanilla whey protein powder (such as Designer Whey)
- [ ] 1 bottle sriracha hot sauce (such as Tuong Ot)

BEVERAGE

- [ ] 2 bottles red wine

PRODUCE

- [ ] 14 Ruby Red grapefruits
- [ ] 2 pints fresh broccoli florets
- [ ] 2 small containers hummus (look for 50 calories per serving, such as Athenos)
- [ ] 4 bunches Tuscan kale
- [ ] 2 bunches curly kale
- [ ] 2 pints diced carrots
- [ ] 4 large cucumbers
- [ ] 6 Granny Smith apples
- [ ] 2 fresh pomegranates or 2 small containers of fresh pomegranate seeds
- [ ] 2 underripe bananas
- [ ] 2 small bags cleaned green beans
- [ ] 18 lemons
- [ ] 2 small papayas or 1 papaya
- [ ] 4 pints mild pico de gallo (such as Ready Pac)
- [ ] 2 pints spicy pico de gallo (such as Ready Pac)
- [ ] 2 bunches cilantro
- [ ] 4 pints cherry tomatoes
- [ ] 2 small jars kimchi
- [ ] 2 bunches mint
- [ ] 2 bunches basil
- [ ] 2 bags broccoli slaw (such as Dole)
- [ ] 2 medium rutabagas
- [ ] 2 heads iceberg lettuce
- [ ] 2 bags frozen no-sugar-added strawberries
- [ ] 6 cups store-prepared plain cucumber, onion, and cherry tomato salad (find in salad bar section or deli counter at supermarket)
- [ ] 2 bunches fresh dill
- [ ] 2 large bunches bok choy
- [ ] 4 small apples (such as Pink Lady, Gala, or Winesap)
- [ ] 2 heads garlic
- [ ] 2 large zucchinis
- [ ] 2 sweet potatoes
- [ ] 2 pints precut fresh mirepoix (diced onion, carrot, celery—look in produce department)
- [ ] 2 bags cleaned fresh sugar snap peas
- [ ] 2 bags frozen sliced mixed bell peppers and onions (such as Birds Eye Pepper and Onion Stir-Fry)
- [ ] 2 pints fresh raspberries
- [ ] 4 large fresh tomatoes
- [ ] 2 pints store-prepared peeled and cut watermelon
- [ ] 2 bunches celery hearts
- [ ] 2 pints (fresh packed) grapefruit sections

- ☐ 2 medium fennel bulbs
- ☐ 2 pints fresh chopped vegetable medley (such as Salad Confetti by Ready Pac)
- ☐ 2 heads butter lettuce
- ☐ 2 bags frozen broccoli florets
- ☐ 4 underripe bananas
- ☐ 4 avocados

DAIRY, EGGS, BREAD

- ☐ Two 35-ounce containers plus two 6-ounce containers fat-free Greek yogurt (such as Fage Total 0%)
- ☐ 4 containers (170g each) sugar-free, fat-free, banana-flavored yogurt (such as Dannon Light & Fit)
- ☐ 2 small containers nonfat cottage cheese (such as Friendship)
- ☐ 2 bottles liquid sugar-free vanilla creamer (such as Coffee-Mate)
- ☐ 2 pints egg whites
- ☐ 6 blocks 75% reduced-fat cheddar cheese (such as Cabot)
- ☐ 1 gallon unsweetened vanilla almond milk (such as Silk)
- ☐ 4 containers sugar-free reduced-calorie vanilla pudding cups (such as Jell-O)
- ☐ 2 pints egg replacement (such as Egg Beaters)
- ☐ 2 packages fat-free American cheese (such as Kraft)

- ☐ 2 packages light whole wheat hamburger buns (such as Sara Lee Delightful Wheat)

PROTEIN

- ☐ 36 ounces store-bought roasted turkey breast, skin removed, sliced ¼ inch thick at deli
- ☐ 20 ounces store-prepared boiled shrimp, shells removed
- ☐ Eight 4-ounce boneless, skinless chicken breast cutlets
- ☐ Two 8-ounce cans sockeye salmon
- ☐ 12 ounces 96% lean ground beef (such as Laura's Lean)
- ☐ 2 packs turkey bacon (such as Butterball Everyday Thin & Crispy)
- ☐ 3 store-roasted chickens
- ☐ 10 ounces pork tenderloin
- ☐ 16 ounces salmon filet (wild sockeye, Chinook, or king is preferable)
- ☐ 2 small cans water-packed no-added-salt light tuna, drained (such as Sustainable Seas)
- ☐ 12 ounces beef tenderloin, well trimmed
- ☐ 2 boxes turkey breakfast sausage patties (such as Bob Evans)

DRY GOODS/PANTRY

- ☐ 1 canister psyllium husk powder
- ☐ 1 canister fiber powder (such as ReNew Life Triple Fiber)

- [ ] 1 canister protein powder (such as Daily Benefit)
- [ ] 1 pound dark unsweetened cocoa powder (such as Hershey's Special Dark)
- [ ] 4 ounces shelled, unsalted pumpkin seeds
- [ ] 2 boxes stevia (such as Stevia In The Raw)
- [ ] Two 11-ounce boxes unsweetened natural coconut water (such as ZICO)
- [ ] Two 24-ounce bags unflavored egg-white powder (such as Jay Robb)
- [ ] 2 pouches poultry gravy mix (such as Knorr Roasted Chicken)
- [ ] 4 ounces no-sugar-added dried cranberries
- [ ] 2 boxes black tea (such as Lipton)
- [ ] 2 boxes green tea (such as sencha)
- [ ] 10 boxes monk fruit extract (such as Monk Fruit In The Raw, 40-count box)
- [ ] 4 cans olive oil spray (such as Pam)
- [ ] 4 packages instant sugar-free banana cream or vanilla pudding mix (such as Jell-O)
- [ ] 4 packages instant sugar-free vanilla pudding mix (such as Jell-O)
- [ ] 2 bags (32g) freeze-dried blueberries (such as Trader Joe's)
- [ ] 1 bottle raw agave nectar
- [ ] 2 bottles calorie-free pancake syrup (such as Walden Farms)
- [ ] 2 ounces shelled black walnuts
- [ ] 2 canisters vanilla whey protein powder (such as Designer Whey)
- [ ] 4 bottles reduced-sodium sugar-free teriyaki sauce (such as Seal Sama)
- [ ] 1 bottle toasted sesame seeds
- [ ] Four 6-ounce bags shirataki rice (such as Miracle Noodle—substitute a different shirataki product and chop it up if the rice cut is not available)
- [ ] 32 ounces shirataki fettuccine (substitute spaghetti if fettuccine not available)
- [ ] 1 box unsalted beef stock (such as Kitchen Basics)
- [ ] 2 cans 98% fat-free cream of mushroom soup (such as Campbell's)
- [ ] 4 bags tofu shirataki macaroni (substitute another shirataki noodle cut if needed)
- [ ] 2½ boxes instant sugar-free chocolate pudding (such as Jell-O)
- [ ] 2 bags organic fat-free milk powder (such as Organic Valley)
- [ ] 2 bags (8.29 ounces) zero-calorie all-natural sweetener (such as Lakanto)
- [ ] 1 canister cinnamon powder
- [ ] 1 canister ginger powder

- ☐ 1 canister crushed red pepper flakes
- ☐ 1 canister cayenne pepper
- ☐ 1 canister seafood seasoning (such as Old Bay)
- ☐ 2 quarts fat-free, unsalted chicken stock or broth (such as Kitchen Basics or Swanson's)
- ☐ 1 box salt-free vegetable bouillon cubes (such as Rapunzel)
- ☐ Six 8-ounce bags shirataki spaghetti
- ☐ 1 canister no-added-salt-or-sugar wasabi powder (such as Eden)
- ☐ 1 can no-added-salt-or-sugar whole peeled plum tomatoes
- ☐ 2 cans reduced-sodium white cannellini beans (such as Eden)
- ☐ Six 6-ounce sugar-free reduced-calorie vanilla pudding cups (such as Jell-O)

- ☐ 1 bottle reduced-sugar ketchup (such as Heinz)
- ☐ 1 bottle red wine vinegar
- ☐ 1 bottle liquid smoke
- ☐ 1 jar prepared horseradish
- ☐ 1 bottle bitters
- ☐ 1 bottle all-natural or pure vanilla extract
- ☐ 1 jar capers
- ☐ 2 envelopes instant brown gravy (such as Knorr)
- ☐ 2 small bags xanthan gum (such as Bob's Red Mill)
- ☐ 8 ounces unsalted almonds
- ☐ 1 bottle no-added-sugar pickled ginger (such as Eden)
- ☐ 1 bottle sriracha hot sauce (such as Tuong Ot)

BEVERAGE

- ☐ 2 bottles red wine

PRODUCE

- ☐ 14 Ruby Red grapefruits
- ☐ 4 bunches curly kale
- ☐ 2 bags broccoli slaw (such as Dole)
- ☐ 2 pints fresh broccoli florets
- ☐ 2 pints chopped carrots (check produce department or salad bar)
- ☐ 2 large cucumbers
- ☐ 4 Granny Smith apples
- ☐ 2 bags frozen sliced mixed bell peppers and onions (such as Birds Eye Pepper and Onion Stir-Fry)
- ☐ 20 lemons
- ☐ 2 bunches basil
- ☐ 2 bags no-sugar-added frozen strawberries
- ☐ 2 bunches cilantro
- ☐ 2 pints spicy store-bought pico de gallo (such as Ready Pac)
- ☐ 4 pints mild store-bought pico de gallo (such as Ready Pac)
- ☐ 2 pints fresh strawberries
- ☐ 2 heads garlic
- ☐ 2 large zucchinis
- ☐ 2 bags (at least 4 cups) fresh cleaned sugar snap peas
- ☐ 2 medium rutabagas
- ☐ 2 pints fresh raspberries
- ☐ 4 small apples (such as Pink Lady, Gala, or Winesap)
- ☐ 4 cups store-prepared plain raw vegetable mix (broccoli, cauliflower, peppers, etc.)
- ☐ 4 pints cherry tomatoes
- ☐ 4 heads iceberg lettuce
- ☐ 2 large bunches bok choy
- ☐ 2 large sweet potatoes
- ☐ 6 cups store-prepared plain cucumber, onion, and cherry tomato salad (find in salad bar section or deli counter at supermarket)
- ☐ 2 bunches fresh dill
- ☐ 4 underripe bananas
- ☐ 2 pints fresh diced tricolor peppers (such as Ready Pac, or you can use frozen)
- ☐ 2 pints fresh diced onions and celery (such as Ready Pac)
- ☐ 2 small containers hummus (look for 50 calories per serving, such as Athenos)
- ☐ 2 bags frozen broccoli florets
- ☐ 2 bags frozen brown and wild rice mix (such as Birds Eye Steamfresh)
- ☐ 2 fennel bulbs
- ☐ 2 pints store-prepared fresh grapefruit sections
- ☐ 6 avocados

DAIRY, EGGS, BREAD

- ☐ 2 bottles liquid sugar-free vanilla coffee creamer (such as Coffee-mate)

- ☐ 2 pints egg whites

- ☐ 6 blocks 75% reduced-fat cheddar cheese (such as Cabot)

- ☐ 1 gallon unsweetened vanilla almond milk (such as Silk)

- ☐ Two 35-ounce containers plus two 17-ounce containers fat-free Greek yogurt (such as Fage Total 0%)

- ☐ 4 containers (170g each) sugar-free, fat-free, banana-flavored yogurt (such as Dannon Light & Fit)

- ☐ 2 small chunks Pecorino Romano

- ☐ 2 pints fat-free milk

- ☐ Six 6-ounce sugar-free reduced-calorie vanilla pudding cups (such as Jell-O)

- ☐ 2 pints egg replacement (such as Egg Beaters)

- ☐ 2 packages fat-free American cheese (such as Kraft)

- ☐ 2 packages light whole wheat hamburger buns (such as Sara Lee Delightful Wheat)

PROTEIN

- ☐ 2 store-roasted chickens

- ☐ 2 pounds turkey breast, sliced ¼ inch thick at deli

- ☐ Eight 4-ounce boneless, skinless chicken cutlets

- ☐ 24 ounces store-prepared boiled shrimp, shells removed

- ☐ 2 packs turkey bacon (such as Butterball Everyday Thin & Crispy)

- ☐ 2 small cans water-packed salmon filet (wild sockeye, Chinook, or king is preferable)

- ☐ 4 dozen littleneck clams with their juice, shucked and chopped by fishmonger (call ahead so the clams are ready when you arrive!)

- ☐ 12 ounces well-trimmed beef tenderloin

- ☐ 2 boxes turkey breakfast sausage patties (such as Bob Evans)

DRY GOODS/PANTRY

- ☐ 1 canister cinnamon powder

- ☐ 1 canister ginger powder

- ☐ 1 bag (8.29 ounces) zero-calorie all-natural sweetener (such as Lakanto)

- ☐ 10 boxes monk fruit extract (such as Monk Fruit In The Raw, 40-count box)

- ☐ 2 boxes black tea (such as Lipton)

- ☐ 2 boxes green tea (such as sencha)

- ☐ 1 canister psyllium husk powder

- ☐ 1 canister fiber powder (such as ReNew Life Triple Fiber)

- ☐ 1 canister protein powder (such as Daily Benefit)
- ☐ 1 pound dark unsweetened cocoa powder (such as Hershey's Special Dark)
- ☐ Two 24-ounce bag unflavored egg-white powder (such as Jay Robb)
- ☐ 2 packages plain air-popped popcorn
- ☐ 1 small canister cayenne pepper
- ☐ 4 cans olive oil spray (such as Pam)
- ☐ 4 bottles reduced-sodium sugar-free teriyaki sauce (such as Seal Sama)
- ☐ 1 bottle pickled cherry peppers
- ☐ 4 bags tofu shirataki spaghetti
- ☐ 2 packages instant sugar-free banana cream or vanilla pudding (such as Jell-O)
- ☐ 2 packages instant sugar-free vanilla pudding (such as Jell-O)
- ☐ 16 ounces shirataki spaghetti
- ☐ 1 canister crushed red pepper flakes
- ☐ 1 jar no-added-salt peanut butter (such as Smucker's Natural)
- ☐ 1 canister red curry paste
- ☐ 2 bags organic fat-free milk powder (such as Organic Valley)
- ☐ 1 bottle red wine vinegar
- ☐ 1 bottle liquid smoke
- ☐ 1 bottle reduced-sugar ketchup (such as Heinz)
- ☐ 1 bottle almond extract
- ☐ 1 canister vanilla whey protein powder (such as Designer Whey)
- ☐ 2 packs original, small-size, low-carb tortillas (such as La Tortilla Factory)
- ☐ 1 bottle raw agave nectar
- ☐ 1 canister no-added-salt-or-sugar wasabi powder (such as Eden)
- ☐ 1 canister toasted sesame seeds
- ☐ 1 bag xanthan gum (such as Bob's Red Mill)
- ☐ 32 ounces shirataki fettuccine (substitute shirataki spaghetti if fettuccine unavailable)
- ☐ 16 ounces shirataki spaghetti
- ☐ 2 bags (32g) no-sugar-added freeze-dried blueberries (such as Trader Joe's)
- ☐ 1 bottle calorie-free pancake syrup (such as Walden Farms)
- ☐ 2 ounces shelled black walnuts
- ☐ Four 6-ounce bags shirataki rice (such as Miracle Noodle—substitute a different shirataki product and chop it up if the rice cut is unavailable)
- ☐ 1 canister seafood seasoning (such as Old Bay)
- ☐ 1 box stevia powder (such as Stevia In The Raw)
- ☐ Two 11-ounce container natural coconut water (such as ZICO)
- ☐ 2 bottles coconut nectar

- ☐ 1 bag freeze-dried strawberries
- ☐ 2 sleeves unsalted brown rice cakes (such as Lundberg)
- ☐ 2 small boxes no-sugar-or-salt-added chopped tomatoes (such as Pomi)
- ☐ 1 canister garlic flakes (such as Frontier)
- ☐ 2 envelopes instant brown gravy (such as Knorr)
- ☐ 1 bottle all-natural or pure vanilla extract
- ☐ 1 canister salt-free adobo powder
- ☐ 2 cans reduced-sodium black beans
- ☐ 2 bags trimmed green beans
- ☐ 1 bottle sriracha hot sauce (such as Tuong Ot)

BEVERAGE

- ☐ 2 bottles red wine

PRODUCE

- [ ] 14 large Ruby Red grapefruits
- [ ] 4 small apples (such as Pink Lady, Gala, or Winesap)
- [ ] 4 large bunches Tuscan kale
- [ ] 2 pints precut carrots (look in produce or salad bar)
- [ ] 2 large cucumbers
- [ ] 6 Granny Smith apples
- [ ] 6 pints cherry tomatoes
- [ ] 4 bunches curly kale
- [ ] 2 fresh pomegranates or 2 small containers pomegranate seeds
- [ ] 2 bags fresh cleaned sugar snap peas
- [ ] 2 bags frozen sliced mixed bell peppers and onions (such as Birds Eye Pepper and Onion Stir-Fry)
- [ ] 2 bunches basil
- [ ] 2 pints fresh strawberries
- [ ] 2 pints fresh raspberries
- [ ] 2 bags broccoli slaw (such as Dole)
- [ ] 2 small papayas or 1 papaya
- [ ] 2 pints spicy store-bought pico de gallo (such as Ready Pac)
- [ ] 4 pints mild store-bought pico de gallo (such as Ready Pac)
- [ ] 2 pints fresh broccoli florets
- [ ] 2 pints store-prepared raw, plain vegetable mix (broccoli, cauliflower, peppers, etc.)
- [ ] 2 bunches cilantro
- [ ] 2 small containers hummus (look for 50 calories per serving, such as Athenos)
- [ ] 2 heads garlic
- [ ] 2 sweet potatoes
- [ ] 2 pints precut fresh mirepoix (diced onion, carrot, celery— look in produce department)
- [ ] 2 pints fresh chopped vegetable medley (such as Salad Confetti by Ready Pac)
- [ ] 2 heads butter lettuce
- [ ] 4 underripe bananas
- [ ] 4 heads iceberg lettuce
- [ ] 2 bags frozen brown and wild rice mix (such as Birds Eye Steamfresh)
- [ ] 4 avocados

DAIRY, EGGS, BREAD

- [ ] 6 blocks 75% reduced-fat cheddar cheese (such as Cabot)
- [ ] Two 35-ounce containers plus two 6-ounce containers fat-free Greek yogurt (such as Fage Total 0%)
- [ ] 2 quarts unsweetened vanilla almond milk (such as Silk)

- ☐ 2 small containers nonfat cottage cheese (such as Friendship)
- ☐ 2 bottles liquid sugar-free vanilla creamer (such as Coffee-Mate)
- ☐ Six 6-ounce sugar-free reduced-calorie vanilla pudding cups (such as Jell-O)
- ☐ 2 pints egg whites
- ☐ 4 containers (170g each) sugar-free, fat-free, banana-flavored yogurt (such as Dannon Light & Fit)
- ☐ 2 pints egg replacement (such as Egg Beaters)
- ☐ 2 packages fat free American cheese (such as Kraft)
- ☐ 2 packages light whole wheat hamburger buns (such as Sara Lee Delightful Wheat)

PROTEIN

- ☐ 48 ounces store-bought roasted turkey breast, skin removed, sliced ¼ inch thick at deli
- ☐ 2 store-roasted chicken
- ☐ 24 ounces store-prepared boiled shrimp, shells removed
- ☐ 10 ounces pork tenderloin, cut into 16 medallions
- ☐ 12 ounces 96% lean ground beef (such as Laura's Lean)
- ☐ 2 cans water-packed no-added-salt light tuna, drained (such as Sustainable Seas)
- ☐ 12 ounces well-trimmed beef tenderloin

- ☐ 2 bags frozen broccoli florets
- ☐ 2 boxes turkey breakfast sausage patties (such as Bob Evans)

DRY GOODS/PANTRY

- ☐ 1 canister cinnamon powder
- ☐ 1 canister ginger powder
- ☐ 2 bags (8.29 ounces) zero-calorie all-natural sweetener (such as Lakanto)
- ☐ 10 boxes monk fruit extract (such as Monk Fruit In The Raw, 40-count box)
- ☐ 2 boxes black tea (such as Lipton)
- ☐ 2 boxes green tea (such as sencha)
- ☐ 1 canister psyllium husk powder
- ☐ 1 canister fiber powder (such as ReNew Life Triple Fiber)
- ☐ 1 canister protein powder (such as Daily Benefit)
- ☐ 1 pound dark unsweetened cocoa powder (such as Hershey's Special Dark)
- ☐ Two 24-ounce bags unflavored egg-white powder (such as Jay Robb)
- ☐ 1 bottle red wine vinegar
- ☐ 2 ounces shelled, unsalted pumpkin seeds
- ☐ 1 canister no-added-salt-or-sugar wasabi powder (such as Eden)
- ☐ 1 canister crushed red pepper flakes

- ❏ 1 jar no-added-sugar-or-salt peanut butter (such as Kraft)
- ❏ 1 canister no-added-sugar red curry paste
- ❏ 32 ounces shirataki spaghetti noodles
- ❏ 1 bottle raw agave nectar
- ❏ 1 bag xanthan gum (such as Bob's Red Mill)
- ❏ 4 bags (32g) no-sugar-added freeze-dried blueberries (such as Trader Joe's)
- ❏ 2 bottles calorie-free pancake syrup (such as Walden Farms)
- ❏ 2 ounces shelled black walnuts
- ❏ 4 bottles reduced-sodium sugar-free teriyaki sauce (such as Seal Sama)
- ❏ 1 jar pickled cherry peppers
- ❏ 1 bottle almond extract
- ❏ 2 boxes instant sugar-free vanilla pudding (such as Jell-O)
- ❏ 2 boxes instant sugar-free banana cream pudding (such as Jell-O)
- ❏ 1 canister vanilla whey protein powder (such as Designer Whey)
- ❏ 2 envelopes poultry gravy mix (such as Knorr Roasted Chicken)
- ❏ 1 bag no-sugar-added dried cranberries
- ❏ 4 packets air-popped popcorn

- ❏ 2 small cans no-added-salt-or-sugar whole peeled plum tomatoes
- ❏ 2 small cans drained reduced-sodium white cannellini beans (such as Eden)
- ❏ 4 cans olive oil spray (such as Pam)
- ❏ 2 small bags organic fat-free milk powder (such as Organic Valley)
- ❏ 2 boxes instant sugar-free chocolate pudding (such as Jell-O)
- ❏ 1 canister seafood seasoning (such as Old Bay)
- ❏ 1 canister sweet smoked paprika
- ❏ 2 quarts fat-free unsalted chicken stock or broth (such as Kitchen Basics or Swanson's)
- ❏ 2 bags (produce) or cans ready-to-eat cooked lentils (such as Melissa's or Eden)
- ❏ 2 boxes instant sugar-free banana cream pudding (such as Jell-O)
- ❏ Two 11.25-ounce box unsalted beef stock (such as Kitchen Basics)
- ❏ 2 small cans 98% fat-free cream of mushroom soup (such as Campbell's)
- ❏ Four 8-ounce bags tofu shirataki macaroni (substitute another shirataki noodle cut if needed)
- ❏ 1 jar brined capers
- ❏ 1 box stevia (such as Stevia In The Raw)

- [ ] Two 11-ounce boxes unsweetened natural coconut water (such as ZICO)

- [ ] 1 bottle red wine vinegar

- [ ] 2 packs original, small-size, low-carb tortillas (such as La Tortilla Factory)

- [ ] 1 bottle all-natural or pure vanilla extract

- [ ] 2 cans reduced-sodium black beans (such as Bush's)

- [ ] 1 canister salt-free adobo powder

- [ ] Four 6-ounce bags shirataki rice (such as Miracle Noodle—substitute a different shirataki product and chop it up if the rice cut is unavailable)

- [ ] 2 envelopes instant brown gravy (such as Knorr)

- [ ] 1 bottle sriracha hot sauce (such as Tuong Ot)

BEVERAGE

- [ ] 2 bottles red wine

CHAPTER 6

Rocco's Pound a Day Diet Recipes

MY PHILOSOPHY is that the best way to shed pounds is to learn to eat for pleasure and enjoy the foods you eat. The truth is, the more pleasure you get from food, the less food you'll need to feel satisfied. Most of us eat so fast that we really don't have time to taste the food we eat or to allow our bodies to tell us we're full.

Be prepared—and pleased—to see some of your favorite foods! Eating our favorite foods—when I've reengineered them as healthy low-calorie versions like these—allows us to feel in control and allows us to truly enjoy eating.

You'll use these recipes during the twenty-eight days of the diet, and on the maintenance plan—but you can use them anytime in the future as well. The recipes are full of flavor, yet low in calories and bad fats and high in fruits and veggies. They're also low in carbs and high in protein, which studies have shown can be an effective pattern for healthy weight loss.

In my earlier *Now Eat This!* series of diet and healthy eating books, I've included before-and-after fat and calorie counts. I'm doing that here, too, to show you how you and I can reengineer some of your favorite comfort foods with a few smart tweaks, so they can deliver the same satisfaction per bite, with significantly fewer calories!

These are some of my fastest, easiest recipes ever.

Lots of them have five ingredients or less and take five minutes or less to prepare. Breakfast items are fast, too, to help you get out the door without a fuss!

To make this super-easy for you, if you absolutely don't have any time to cook (and I think you should make the time), I've listed ready-made substitutions.

You'll see that most recipes serve four. To prepare fewer servings, like one or two, simply divide the recipe amounts accordingly. If you have family members who aren't on the diet, they can have additional servings and eat other things during the day. If you like to cook ahead, you can cook two days' worth of meals, keep them in the fridge, and warm them up when you want.

The food is delicious, but no two palates are alike, so feel free to customize by seasoning your food with zero-calorie-impact seasonings like lemon or lime juice, salt, pepper, Tabasco, all spices, all herbs, vinegars, garlic powder, onion powder, and horseradish. Make your food taste good to your palate.

You'll see that there's a LOT of food; you should not be hungry.

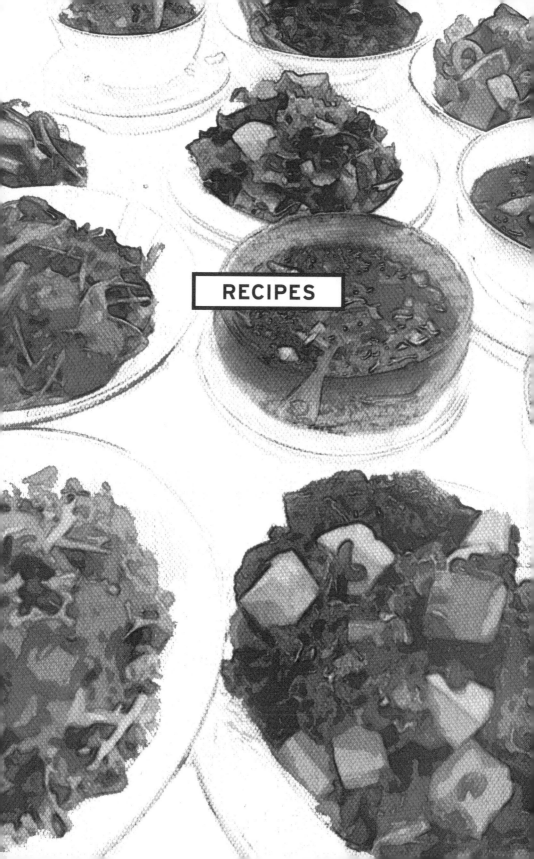

RECIPES

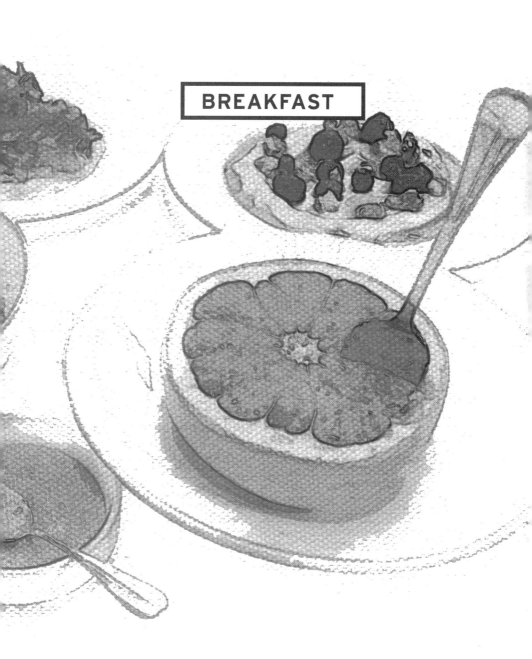

BREAKFAST

PROTEIN-PACKED BREAKFAST SANDWICH

C | 188
F | 3g

HAVE AN AMERICAN CLASSIC with a flavorful and super-healthy twist.

Yield:	Prep time:	Cooking time:
4 servings	about 1 minute	about 5 minutes

Ingredients:

Olive oil cooking spray (such as Pam)

4   lean turkey breakfast sausage patties (such as Bob Evans)

4   slices fat-free American cheese (such as Kraft)

4   light whole-wheat hamburger buns (such as Sara Lee Delightful Wheat)

1   cup egg replacement (such as Egg Beaters)

Salt and freshly ground pepper to taste

2   tablespoons sriracha (such as Tuong Ot)

Method:

1. *Spray* a large nonstick skillet with 1 second of cooking spray and place over medium-high heat. Once the skillet is hot, add the sausage patties and *brown* on one side, about 1 minute. *Flip* each patty and brown the other side, about another minute. Remove the patties from the skillet, *place* a piece of cheese over each one, and set aside in a warm place. Put the buns in the skillet, cut side down, to *toast*, about 30 seconds. Place one bun each on four separate plates.

2. *Add* the egg replacement to the skillet and *cook* over medium-high heat until cooked through; season with salt and pepper. Evenly *divide* the cooked eggs among the bottom halves of the hamburger buns. Place the sausage patties on the top of each of the egg layers, then *top* each patty with ½ tablespoon of sriracha and serve.

Per serving:

188 calories, 3g fat (.5g sat), 23mg cholesterol, 885mg sodium, 18.5g carbohydrate, 6.5g fiber, 19.5g protein

Nutrient content claims:

Reduced fat / Low fat / Low saturated fat / High fiber / High protein / Trans fat free

---

Recommended ready-made version:
Weight Watchers Smart Ones
Calories: 230 / Fat: 8g

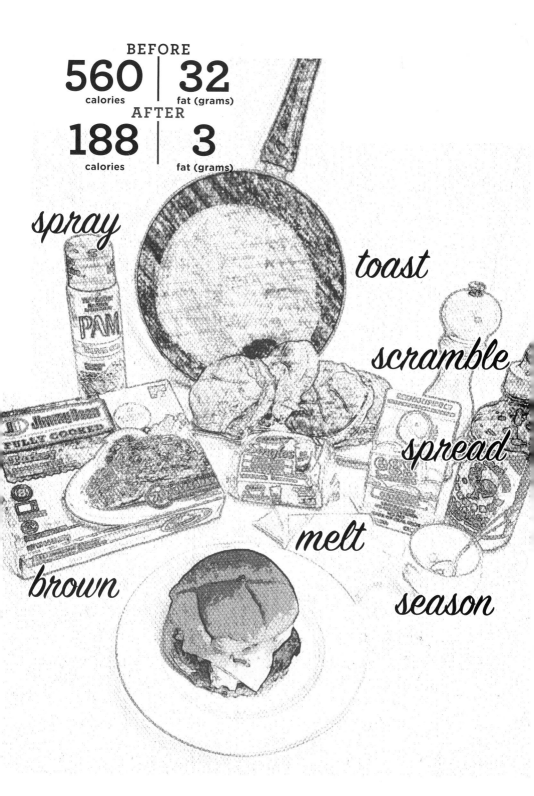

BEFORE

560 calories | 32 fat (grams)

AFTER

188 calories | 3 fat (grams)

spray

toast

scramble

spread

melt

brown

season

87

PROTEIN-PACKED BREAKFAST SANDWICH

ALL-DAY EGG-WHITE OMELET WITH PICO DE GALLO

C | 70
F | 1g

THIS SUPER-QUICK meal replacement is not only filling but can be tailored to satisfy any flavor craving you may have. Think of it like a super-fast pizza without borders that you can use to provide your favorite flavor combinations.

Yield:	Prep time:	Cooking time:
4 servings	about 3 minutes	about 5 minutes

Ingredients:

Olive oil cooking spray (such as Pam)

1 cup egg whites (or prepared 100% egg whites, such as Egg Beaters)

Salt and freshly ground black pepper

2 ounces 75% reduced-fat cheddar cheese, shredded (such as Cabot)

1/2 cup ready-made pico de gallo or tomato salsa (such as Ready Pac)

1/2 cup fresh cilantro sprigs

Method:

1. *Spray* a microwave-safe 6-inch plate (inside dimension) with 1 second of cooking spray and *pour* 1/4 cup of the egg whites directly onto the plate. *Season* lightly with salt and pepper, place in the microwave, and cook on high until the eggs are just beginning to set up and become cooked, about 1 minute. Remove the plate from the microwave, *sprinkle* on one-quarter of the cheese, and continue to cook on high until the eggs are cooked and the cheese is melted, about another minute. Repeat with the remaining egg whites.

2. Remove the last plate from the microwave. *Spoon* one-quarter of the pico de gallo over each plate, *top* each with one-quarter of the cilantro, and serve.

Tips:

• Sneak an ounce of steamed shrimp on this for an additional 28 calories, less than half a gram of fat, and almost 6 grams of additional protein!

• Use a wider microwave-safe bowl or plate to cook all the eggs at once for a large omelet you can serve family style. Cook the larger plate for 4 to 5 minutes on high.

Per serving:

70 calories, 1g fat (0g sat), 5mg cholesterol, 216mg sodium, 4g carbohydrate, 0g fiber, 11g protein

Nutrient content claims:

Reduced calorie / Low fat / Saturated fat free / Low cholesterol / High protein / Trans fat free / Gluten free

BEFORE

250 | 19
calories | fat (grams)

AFTER

70 | 1
calories | fat (grams)

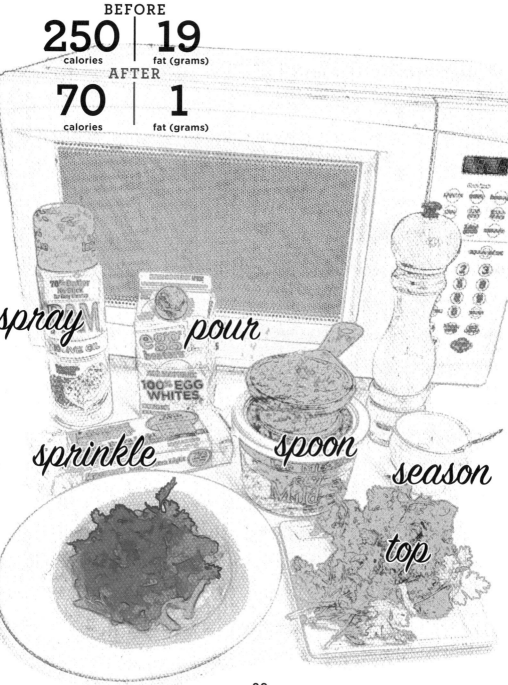

spray

pour

sprinkle

spoon

season

top

89

ALL-DAY EGG-WHITE OMELET WITH PICO DE GALLO

GREEK YOGURT WITH CRUNCHY BLUEBERRY TOPPING

C | 142
F | 4g

THIS SUPER-QUICK meal replacement is not only filling but also packed with wholesome nutrients to keep you moving until your next meal. Walnuts are rich in the omega-3 fat alphalinoleic acid, which improves artery function and promotes bone health, and the blueberries are packed with vitamin C, dietary fiber, and antioxidant activity. While the two give a great textural contrast to the creamy yogurt, combined they offer a wide range of nutrients that will keep you feeling good!

Yield:	Prep time:	Cooking time:
4 servings	about 1 minute	about 2 minute

Ingredients:

2　cups fat-free plain Greek yogurt (such as Fage Total 0%)
4　tablespoons black walnuts, toasted and chopped
1　bag (32g) no-sugar-added freeze-dried blueberries (such as Trader Joe's)
4　tablespoons calorie-free pancake syrup (such as Walden Farms)

Method:

1. *Spoon* the yogurt evenly in four wide dollops in the middle of four small round plates. Evenly *distribute* the walnuts and blueberries over the surface of the yogurt, then *drizzle* each dish with 1 tablespoon of the syrup.

Tip:

• While this is a cool, refreshing dish for warmer weather, you can make a soul-satisfying, belly-warming version for colder days by simply adding the blueberries to the syrup and microwaving for 30 seconds before drizzling over the yogurt. Trust me, it's worth spending the extra 30 seconds!

Per serving:

142 calories, 4g fat (0g sat), 0mg cholesterol, 78mg sodium, 12.75g carbohydrate, 2.25g fiber, 13.5g protein

Nutrient content claims:

Reduced calorie / Reduced fat / Saturated fat free / Cholesterol free / Low sodium / No added sugar / High protein / Gluten free / Trans fat free

Recommended ready-made version:
Fage Total 0% Yogurt with Blueberry 5.3 oz.
Calories: 120 / Fat: 0g

BEFORE

736 | **37**
calories | fat (grams)

AFTER

142 | **4**
calories | fat (grams)

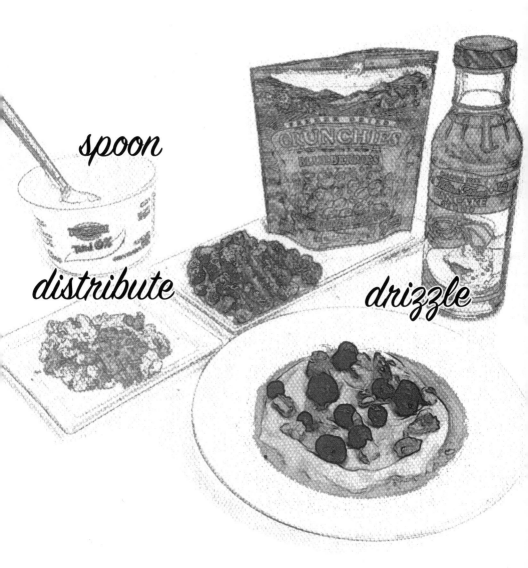

spoon

distribute

drizzle

91

GREEK YOGURT WITH CRUNCHY BLUEBERRY TOPPING

INSTANT OATMEAL WITH PSYCHEDELIC FRUIT CRISPIES

C | 181
F | 3g

IT'S HARD to fit some of our most beloved belly-warming dishes into a healthy profile. Luckily, a bowl of hot oatmeal is not one of them! Yes, I could have just used fresh fruit here, but I am a chef who loves funky textures and using dehydrated fruits, and since the dehydration process happens at such a low temperature, we don't see an increase in the glycemic index.

Yield:	Prep time:	Cooking time:
4 servings	about 1 minute	about 3 minutes

Ingredients:

1	**cup water**
1/2	**teaspoon cinnamon**
4	**packets monk fruit extract (such as Monk Fruit In The Raw)**
2	**cups instant unsweetened oatmeal (such as Quaker)**
1	**cup unsweetened freeze-dried berry mix (such as Crunchies Tropical Fruit)**

Method:

1. *Pour* the water, cinnamon, and monk fruit extract into a medium-sized saucepot and bring to a *boil* over high heat. Turn off the heat, *add* the oatmeal, and *stir* until the water is absorbed, about 1 minute. Pour into four bowls and *sprinkle* each bowl evenly with the berries.

Tip:

• Leave out the berries and save about 30 calories and 1 gram of fat per serving.

Per serving:

181 calories, 3g fat (.75g sat), 0mg cholesterol, 112.5mg sodium, 37g carbohydrate, 5.5g fiber, 6g protein

Nutrient content claims:

Reduced calorie / Low fat / Low saturated fat / Reduced fat / Cholesterol free / Low sodium / No added sugar / Trans fat free

Recommended ready-made version:
San Gennaro Foods Frozen Steel Cut Oatmeal
Calories: 110 / Fat: 3g

BEFORE

1,240 calories | **72** fat (grams)

AFTER

181 calories | **3** fat (grams)

add & stir

pour & boil

sprinkle

INSTANT OATMEAL WITH PSYCHEDELIC FRUIT CRISPIES

APPLE CINNAMON
CRUNCH CEREAL
C | 113
F | 0g

I KNOW it's hard to ditch those sweet cereals, so I've developed this super-quick substitution you can eat if you just can't let go.

Yield:	Prep time:	Cooking time:
4 servings	about 2 minutes	about 3 minutes

Ingredients:

2	cups cold water
3	tablespoons fat-free milk powder (such as Organic Valley)
4	packets monk fruit extract (such as Monk Fruit In The Raw)
	Pinch of salt
3	cups unsweetened puffed brown rice (such as Arrowhead Mills)
½	teaspoon cinnamon
1	cup unsweetened cinnamon apple chips, crushed into small pieces (such as Bare Fruit)

Method:

1. *Combine* the water, milk powder, monk fruit extract, and salt in a small bowl and *whisk* until all the ingredients are completely dissolved, about 30 seconds.

2. *Toss* the puffed rice, cinnamon, and apple chips in a mixing bowl to combine. Pour 1 cup of the puffed rice and apple mixture into each of four bowls, *pour* ½ cup of "milk" into each bowl, and *serve*.

Tip:

- You can mix the apple chips and rice together and keep the mixture in a container with a tight-fitting lid; make it in batches and keep in the pantry for easy use during the week.

Per serving:

113 calories, 0g fat (0g sat), 112.5mg cholesterol, 37.5mg sodium, 26.75g carbohydrate, 2.5 g fiber, 3g protein

Nutrient content claims:

Reduced calorie / Fat free / Saturated fat free / Low sodium / No added sugar / Good source of fiber / Trans fat free / Gluten free

> *Recommended ready-made version:*
> Barbara's Puffins Multigrain
> **Calories: 130 / Fat: 0g**

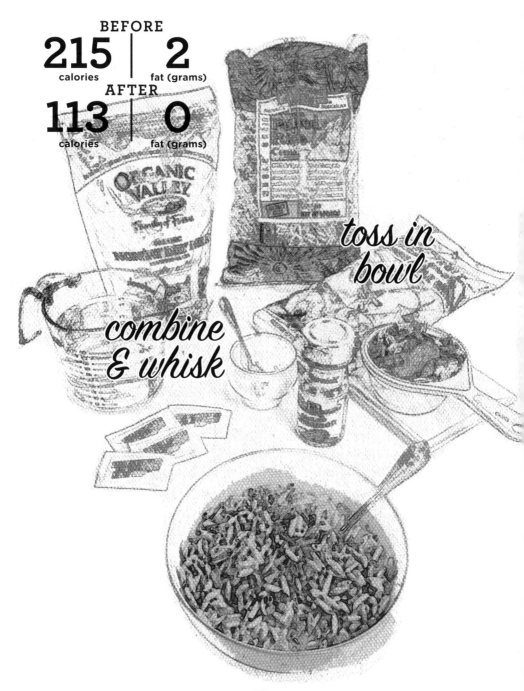

BEFORE

215 calories | **2** fat (grams)

AFTER

113 calories | **0** fat (grams)

combine & whisk

toss in bowl

95

APPLE CINNAMON CRUNCH CEREAL

GRAPEFRUIT WITH ZERO-CALORIE SPICED "SUGAR"

C | 28
F | 0g

THIS QUICK START is a great way to get your palate and body energized. This is a healthy riff on a killer grapefruit preparation made by smothering the fruit in brown sugar and then broiling it until it caramelizes. I love the dish and needed to find a quick replacement. Grapefruit is extremely good for you, high in vitamins A and C; it also has very good levels of the electrolyte potassium, which helps your body counter sodium. The red varieties are even a good source of lycopene, and studies have shown that lycopene protects us from skin damage.

Yield:
4 servings

Prep time:
about 5 minutes

Ingredients:

2   large Ruby Red grapefruits, cut in half crosswise and flesh separated from membrane

1$\frac{1}{2}$ tablespoons large-crystal sugar replacement (such as Lakanto)

$\frac{1}{8}$ teaspoon ginger powder

$\frac{1}{2}$ teaspoon cinnamon powder

Method:

1. *Place* each grapefruit half cut side up in a serving bowl.

2. *Mix* the sugar replacement well with the ginger and cinnamon and *sprinkle* the spiced "sugar" evenly over each grapefruit half. Serve chilled.

Per serving:

28 calories, 0g fat (0g sat), 0mg cholesterol, 0mg sodium, 11g carbohydrate, 2g fiber, 0.5g protein

Nutrient content claims:

Low calorie / Fat free / Saturated fat free / Cholesterol free / Sodium free / No added sugar / Trans fat free / Gluten free

---

Recommended ready-made version:
Store-bought prepared grapefruit segments, $\frac{1}{4}$ cup
Calories: 32 / Fat: 0g

BEFORE

392 | 0.5

calories | fat (grams)

AFTER

28 | 0

calories | fat (grams)

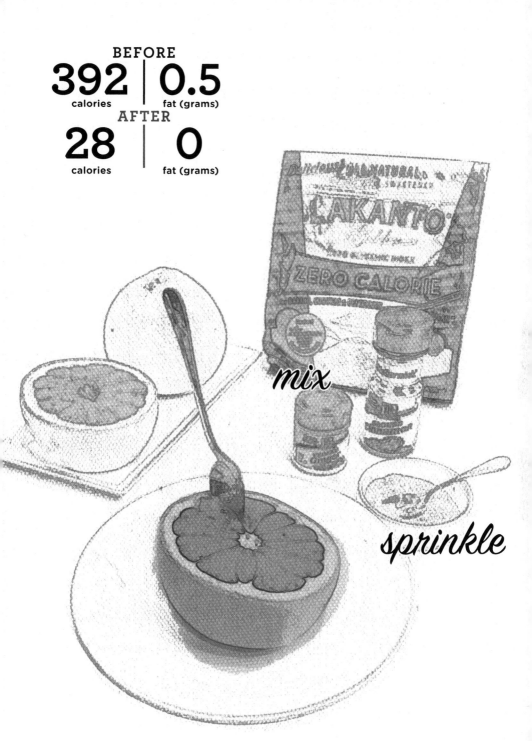

mix

sprinkle

GRAPEFRUIT WITH ZERO-CALORIE SPICED "SUGAR"

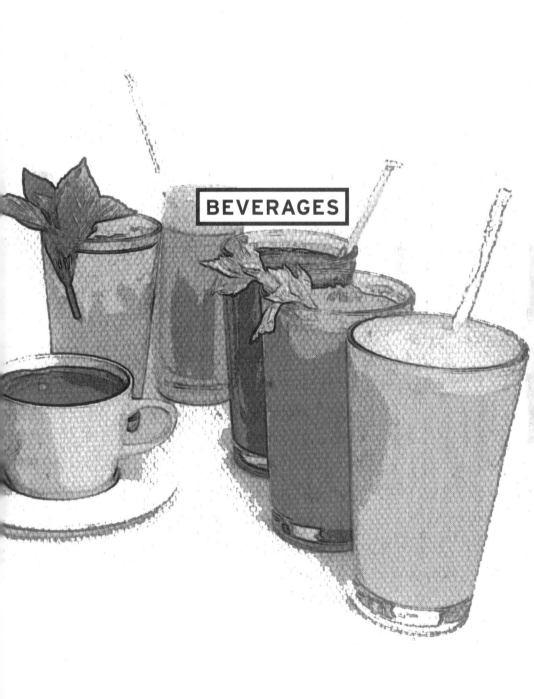

BEVERAGES

BANANA CREAM
SMOOTHIE

C | 103
F | 0g

THIS SUPER-FILLING, very large smoothie gets its body from green (underripe) bananas, part of the wonderful world of resistant starches—meaning that your body processes only a fraction of the carbohydrates found in green bananas, as opposed to ripe ones! If that's not exciting enough, wait until you taste it! My smoothie also gets an extra boost of electrolytes and potassium from the coconut water and protein from the yogurt and egg-white powder.

Yield:	Prep time:	Processing time:
Four 16-ounce servings	about 3 minutes	about 2 minutes

Ingredients:

3   containers (170g each) sugar-free, fat-free banana-flavored yogurt (such as Dannon Light & Fit)

4   packets stevia (such as Stevia In The Raw)

1/2   cup unsweetened plain coconut water (such as ZICO)

1   cup cold water

1   cup sliced slightly underripe banana

3 1/2 cups ice

1   tablespoon egg-white powder (such as Jay Robb)

1/8   teaspoon salt (optional)

Method:

1. Put the yogurt, stevia, coconut water, cold water, and banana in a blender and *blend* until smooth. *Add* half the ice and blend until smooth. *Add* the egg-white powder, salt (if using), and remaining ice and blend until smooth. *Pour* into four cold pint glasses and serve.

Per serving:

103 calories, 0g fat (.043g sat), 2.5mg cholesterol, 74mg sodium, 22g carbohydrate, 1g fiber, 5g protein

Nutrient content claims:

Reduced calorie / Fat free / Saturated fat free / Low cholesterol / Trans fat free / No added sugar / Low sodium

---

Recommended ready-made version:
Pure Protein Banana Cream Shake
Calories: 160 / Fat: 1g

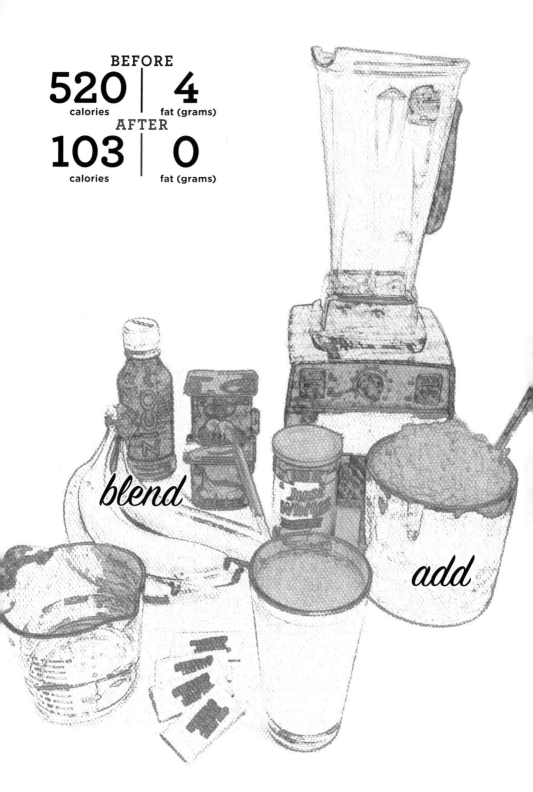

BEFORE

520 | **4**
calories | fat (grams)

AFTER

103 | **0**
calories | fat (grams)

blend

add

BANANA CREAM SMOOTHIE

THE GREEN MONKEY C | 77
F | 0g

I LOVE this recipe because it delivers a jolt of nutrition in a smoothie that fills you up. The base is made with low-calorie-density cucumbers, a little enzyme-rich apple to cover the taste of the greens, and a little natural sweetness from carrots, and I like to use the fast low-calorie thickening power of instant sugar-free pudding.

Yield:	Prep time:	Processing time:
4 servings	about 2 minutes	about 3 minutes

Ingredients:

2   **cups water**

½   **cup carrots, chopped**

2   **cups kale**

2   **cups green cucumbers, skin on, cut into large chunks**

2   **cups Granny Smith apples, skin on, cut into large chunks**

½   **package instant sugar-free banana cream pudding (such as Jell-O)**

2   **cups ice**

4   **packets monk fruit extract (such as Monk Fruit In The Raw; optional)**

Method:

1. *Add* the water and carrots to a blender and *blend* until smooth; *add* the kale, cucumbers, apples, and monk fruit extract (if using) and *blend* until smooth, about 30 more seconds. *Add* the pudding mix and *blend* until thickened, about 30 seconds. *Add* the ice and blend until smooth. Serve.

Tip:

• Use the monk fruit extract if you like things a bit sweeter.

Per serving:

77 calories, 0g fat (0g sat), 0mg cholesterol, 176.5mg sodium, 18g carbohydrate, 2.5g fiber, 2g protein

Nutrient content claims:

Reduced calorie / Fat free / Saturated fat free / Cholesterol free / No added sugar / Good source of fiber / Trans fat free / Gluten free

---

Recommended ready-made version:
Naked Green Machine
Calories: 140 / Fat: 0g

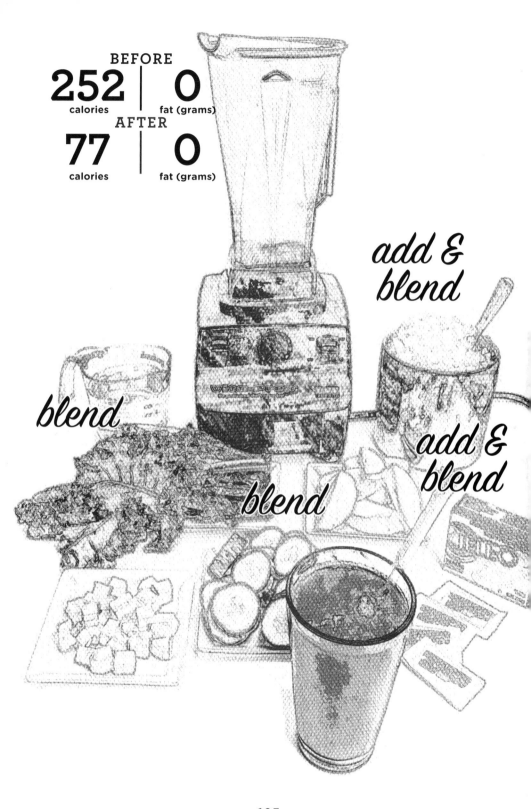

BEFORE

252 | 0
calories | fat (grams)

AFTER

77 | 0
calories | fat (grams)

add & blend

blend

blend

add & blend

SOUTHERN-STYLE SWEET TEA C | 3 · F | 0g

THIS ALL-NATURAL, sugar-free Southern-Style Sweet Tea is something I keep in my refrigerator all summer long. Best thing is that it's a great base to build on: Most tea is healthy and almost calorie free, so knock yourself out! The FDA has determined that anything under 5 calories per serving can be called "calorie free." I hold myself to more specific standards for diet menu calculations, but who would ever think of having a calorie-free sweet tea without artificial sweeteners!

Yield: Four 16-ounce servings	Prep time: about 1 minute	Processing time: about 4 minutes

Ingredients:

- 8 cups cold water
- 6 bags black tea (such as Lipton)
- 1 lemon, zest and juice separate (3 tablespoons juice)
- 16 packets monk fruit extract (such as Monk Fruit In The Raw)
- 4 sprigs mint
  Ice for serving

Method:

1. *Pour* 3 cups of the water into a saucepot with the tea, lemon zest, and monk fruit extract and bring to a *simmer* over high heat. *Pour* the remaining cold water into a pitcher and *strain* the tea into the pitcher with the lemon juice.

2. *Place* 1 mint sprig each in four glasses with ice, *pour* the tea into each glass, and serve.

Tips:

- Use any other natural tea in this recipe for some diversity—I love chamomile, green tea (sencha), hibiscus, and pomegranate.
- Try adding a few sprigs of mint for a fresh touch!
- If you like your tea thicker (from sugar syrup), try adding $1/4$ teaspoon xanthan gum (such as Bob's Red Mill) to the tea and blending on low for 30 seconds. (Xanthan gum's thickening ability varies from brand to brand; I suggest starting with $1/8$ teaspoon to judge the results.)

Per serving:
3 calories, 0g fat (0g sat), 0mg cholesterol, 0mg sodium, 1g carbohydrate, 0.2g fiber, 0.05g protein

Nutrient content claims:
Low calorie / Fat free / Saturated fat free / Cholesterol free / Sodium free / No added sugar / Gluten free / Trans fat free

BEFORE

280 | **0**

calories | fat (grams)

AFTER

3 | **0**

calories | fat (grams)

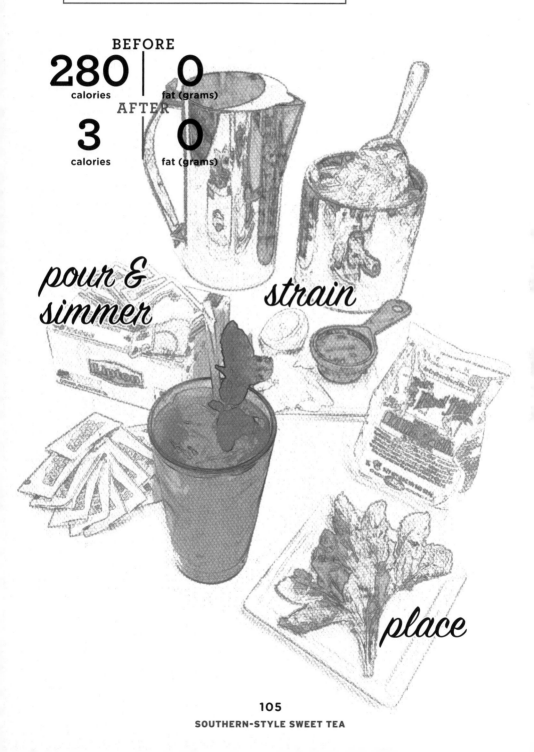

*pour &
simmer*

strain

place

MEXICAN HOT CHOCOLATE

C | 42
F | 0.5g

HERE IS A RECIPE for one of the greatest American indulgences, with a Mexican twist, that won't keep you in that oversized sweater for longer than the weather mandates. This recipe gets great texture from xanthan gum, loses unnecessary calories with skim milk, and provides a metabolism boost with cayenne.

Yield:	Prep time:	Cooking time:
Four 8-ounce servings	about 5 minutes	about 3 minutes

Ingredients:

1	**quart water**
¼	**cup dark unsweetened cocoa powder (such as Hershey's Special Dark)**
½	**teaspoon cinnamon**
4	**tablespoons fat-free milk powder (such as Organic Valley)**
16	**packets monk fruit extract (such as Monk Fruit In The Raw)**
½	**teaspoon xanthan gum (such as Bob's Red Mill)**
	Cayenne pepper to taste
	Salt to taste

Method:

1. Put all the ingredients except for the xanthan gum, cayenne, and salt in a blender and *blend* on medium speed until well mixed. With the blender still running, *add* the gum and *process* until thickened, about 30 seconds. *Add* a tiny bit of cayenne and a pinch of salt and *taste* to see if it's as hot as you like it.

2. *Pour* into four microwave-safe mugs and *cook* on high until hot, about 3 minutes. Serve.

Per serving:
42 calories, 0.5g fat (0g sat), 2mg cholesterol, 108.75mg sodium, 7.8g carbohydrate, 2.2g fiber, 4g protein

Nutrient content claims:
Reduced calorie / Low fat / Saturated fat free / Low cholesterol / Low sodium / No added sugar / Gluten free / Trans fat free

> *Recommended ready-made version:*
> Swiss Miss fat-free hot cocoa
> Calories: 50 / Fat: 0g

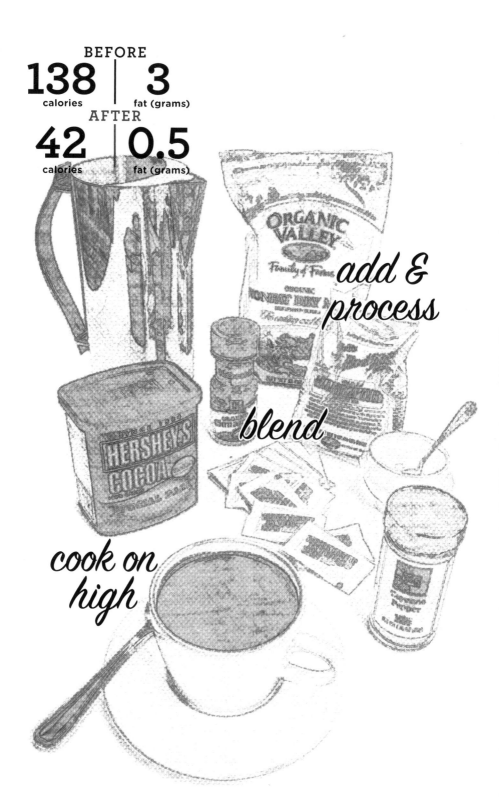

BEFORE
138 calories | **3** fat (grams)

AFTER
42 calories | **0.5** fat (grams)

add & process

blend

cook on high

MEXICAN HOT CHOCOLATE

GREEN TEA WITH LEMON AND BASIL C|4 F|0g

I LOVE SERVING this cold beverage along with refreshing salads and stir-fry dishes. Its complexity is interesting enough to keep you from missing that glass of white wine when you're trimming weight.

| Yield: Four 16-ounce servings | Prep time: about 1 minute | Cooking time: about 4 minutes |

Ingredients:

8 cups cold water
6 bags green tea (such as sencha)
1 lemon, zest and juice separate (3 tablespoons juice)
16 packets monk fruit extract (such as Monk Fruit In The Raw)
1 bunch basil, chopped, with 4 sprigs reserved whole
Ice for serving

Method:

1. *Pour* 3 cups of the water into a saucepot with the tea, lemon zest, monk fruit extract, and chopped basil and bring to a *simmer* over high heat. *Pour* the remaining cold water into a pitcher, *strain* the tea into the pitcher, and *add* the lemon juice.

2. *Place* 1 basil sprig each in four glasses with ice, pour the tea into each glass, and serve.

Tips:

- Use any other natural tea in this recipe for some diversity—I love chamomile, hibiscus, and pomegranate.
- If you like your tea thicker (from sugar syrup), try adding 1/4 teaspoon xanthan gum (such as Bob's Red Mill) to the tea and blending on low for 30 seconds. (Xanthan gum's thickening ability varies from brand to brand; I suggest starting with 1/8 teaspoon to judge the results.)

Per serving:
4 calories, 0g fat (0g sat), 0mg cholesterol, 5.395mg sodium, 5.395g carbohydrate, 0.32g fiber, 0.1975g protein

Nutrient content claims:
Calorie free / Fat free / Saturated fat free / Cholesterol free / Low sodium / No added sugar / Gluten free / Trans fat free

> *Recommended ready-made version:*
> The Tea Nation Iced Green Tea, Jasmine
> Calories: 0 / Fat: 0g

BEFORE

280 | **0**
calories | fat (grams)

AFTER

4 | **0**
calories | fat (grams)

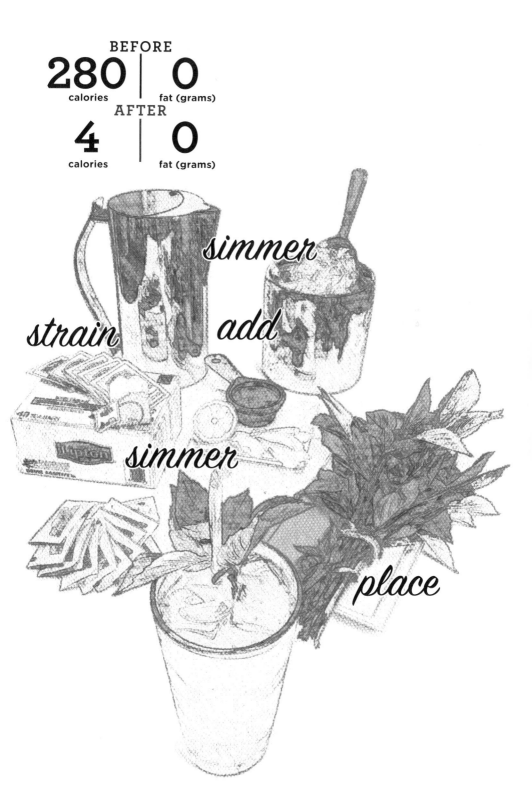

simmer

strain

add

simmer

place

GREEN TEA WITH LEMON AND BASIL

GINGER BOOST PEACH SMOOTHIE

C | 106
F | 7g

A DELICIOUS SMOOTHIE, super-fast.

Yield:	Prep time:	Processing time:
Four 12-ounce servings	about 2 minutes	about 1 minute

Ingredients:

2   cups cold water

4   cups frozen no-added-sugar peaches

2   scoops vanilla whey protein powder (such as Designer Whey)

3/4   teaspoon turmeric

2 1/2   teaspoons grated fresh ginger

1   sugar-free, all-natural lemonade stick (such as Now Real Food Slender Sticks, acai lemonade variety)

2   cups crushed ice or small ice cubes

Method:

1. Put all the ingredients except the ice into a blender and *blend* until smooth, about 30 seconds. Turn off the blender, *add* the ice, and continue to *blend* until smooth, about 30 seconds.

2. *Pour* into 4 pint glasses and serve chilled.

Per serving:

106 calories, 1g fat (.5g sat), 30mg cholesterol, 40.5g sodium, 17.25g carbohydrate, 2.1g fiber, 10.1g protein

Nutrient content claims:

Reduced calorie / Low fat / Low saturated fat / Low sodium / No added sugar / High protein

---

Recommended ready-made version:
SDC Nutrition About Time Peaches and Cream Whey Protein Shake
Calories: 125 / Fat: 0g

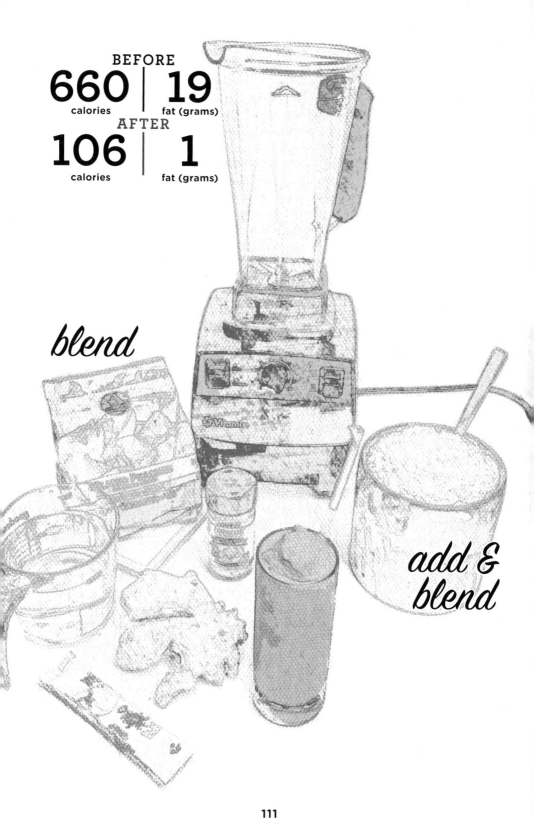

BEFORE

660 | **19**
calories | fat (grams)

AFTER

106 | **1**
calories | fat (grams)

blend

add &
blend

HIGH-PROTEIN CHOCOLATE
BREAKFAST SMOOTHIE

C | 198
F | 2g

THIS SUPER-FILLING, very large smoothie gets your day started with 30 grams of protein delivered in a delicious high-fiber chocolate drink!

Yield:	Prep time:	Processing time:
Four 16-ounce servings	about 3 minutes	about 2 minutes

Ingredients:

6	cups cold water
2	tablespoons psyllium husk powder
2	scoops fiber powder (such as ReNew Life Triple Fiber)
2	scoops protein powder (such as Daily Benefit)
¼	cup plus 2 tablespoons dark unsweetened cocoa powder (such as Hershey's Special Dark)
24	packets monk fruit extract (such as Monk Fruit In the Raw; optional)
4	scoops unflavored egg-white powder (such as Jay Robb)
2	cups crushed ice or small ice cubes

Method:

1. Put the water, psyllium husk powder, and fiber powder in a blender and *blend* on high until smooth and slightly thickened, about 1 ½ minutes. Turn the blender off and *add* the protein powder and cocoa (and monk fruit if using); *blend* until smooth, about 30 seconds, and turn off the blender.

2. *Add* the egg-white powder and *blend* until smooth, about 10 seconds, then *add* the ice and *blend* until smooth, about 30 seconds. Pour the smoothie into 4 pint-sized glasses.

Tip:

- Add a pinch of salt if your diet can afford the sodium—it will really draw out the full flavor of the cocoa.

Per serving:
198 calories, 2g fat (.25g sat), 0mg cholesterol, 488mg sodium, 15g carbohydrate, 8g fiber, 30.75g protein

Nutrient content claims:
Reduced calorie / Low fat / Low saturated fat / Cholesterol free / No added sugar / High fiber / High protein / Gluten free / Trans fat free

---

Recommended ready-made version:
Pure Protein Chocolate Mint
Calories: 160 / Fat: 1.5g

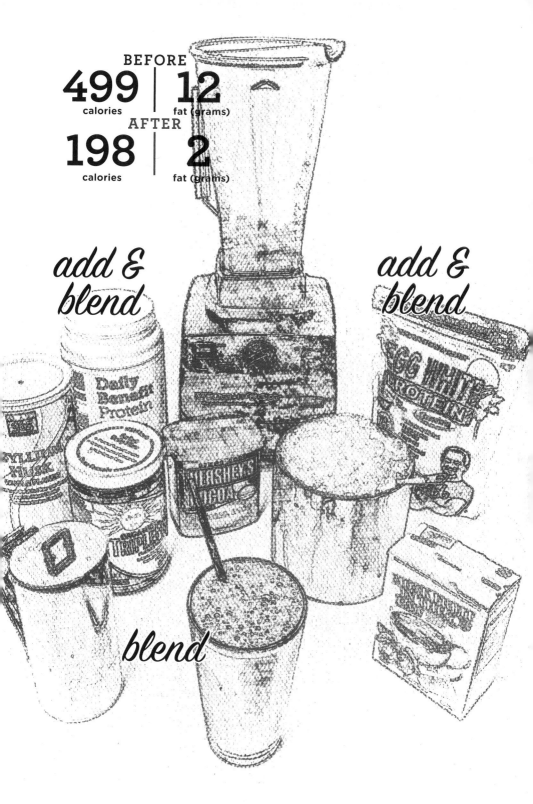

BEFORE
499 | **12**
calories | fat (grams)
AFTER
198 | **2**
calories | fat (grams)

*add &
blend*

*add &
blend*

blend

VIRGIN MARY
C | 46
F | 0g

A GOOD TOOL to have in the recipe belt for the weekends. This low-calorie, large, and refreshing beverage is great for enjoying while socializing with nondieting friends and family. The Bloody Mary is a good cocktail option relative to its sugary cousins, but this *how low can you go* version has so few calories you can enjoy it anytime you like!

Yield:	Prep time:
Four 16-ounce servings	3 minutes

Ingredients:

4   **cups fresh tomatoes**

4   **cups store-bought cut-up watermelon**

¼   **cup fresh lemon juice (check the produce department for ready-squeezed!)**

1   **tablespoon plus 1 teaspoon prepared horseradish**

1   **cup chopped celery, plus 4 inner stalks for garnish**

1   **teaspoon bitters (optional)**

    Ice for serving

Method:

1. *Put* all the ingredients in a blender and *blend* until smooth. *Pour* into 4 pint-sized glasses filled with ice and *garnish* with the celery stalks.

Per serving:

46 calories, 0g fat (0g sat), 1.5mg cholesterol, 44.5mg sodium, 45.5g carbohydrate, 2g fiber, 2g protein

Nutrient content claims:

Reduced calorie / Fat free / Saturated fat free / Cholesterol free / Low sodium / No added sugar / Gluten free / Trans fat free

---

Recommended ready-made version:
Mr. & Mrs. T. Bloody Mary Mix
Calories: 30 / Fat: 0g

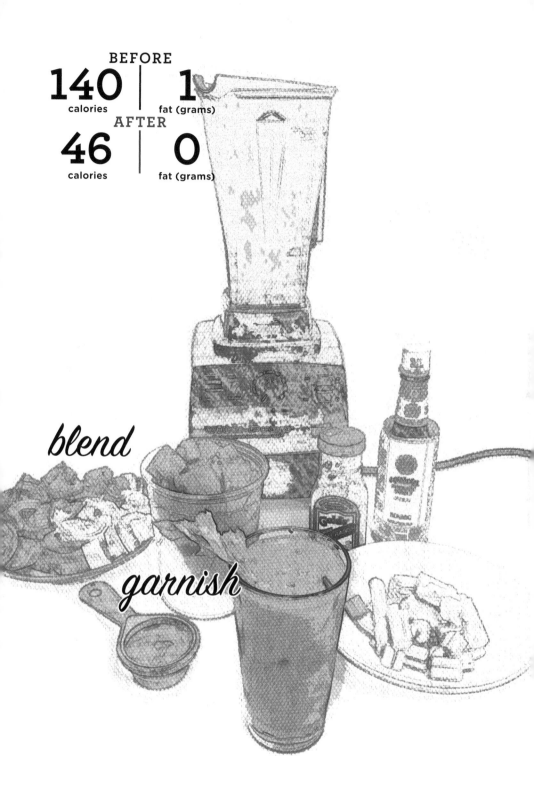

BEFORE
140 calories | 1 fat (grams)

AFTER
46 calories | 0 fat (grams)

blend

garnish

ALMOND MILK SMOOTHIE

C | 84
F | 3g

THIS DELICIOUS SMOOTHIE is a great meal replacement option or a snack to stave off that pesky craving between lunch and dinner.

Yield:	Prep time:	Processing time:
Four 16-ounce servings	about 2 minutes	about 3 minutes

Ingredients:

4   cups unsweetened vanilla almond milk (such as Silk)

¹/₂   teaspoon almond extract

1   scoop vanilla whey protein powder (such as Designer Whey)

3   tablespoons sugar-free instant vanilla pudding (such as Jell-O)

12   packets monk fruit extract (such as Monk Fruit In The Raw)

¹/₄   cup egg-white powder (such as Jay Robb)

2   cups crushed ice or small ice cubes

Method:

1. *Add* the almond milk, almond extract, protein powder, pudding mix, and monk fruit extract in a blender and *blend* on low until well combined, about 20 seconds. *Add* the egg-white powder and *blend* until smooth, about 10 seconds, then *add* the ice and *blend* until smooth, about 30 seconds.

2. *Pour* the smoothie into 4 glasses and serve.

Per serving:

84 calories, 3g fat (0g sat), 5mg cholesterol, 470mg sodium, 5g carbohydrate, 0g fiber, 9.75g protein

Nutrient content claims:

Reduced calorie / Low fat / Saturated fat free / Trans fat free / Low cholesterol / No added sugar / Gluten free

---

Recommended ready-made version:
Medifast French Vanilla Shake
Calories: 110 / Fat: 0.5g

---

355 | **13**
calories | fat (grams)

84 | **3**
calories | fat (grams)

add &
blend

add &
blend

add &
blend

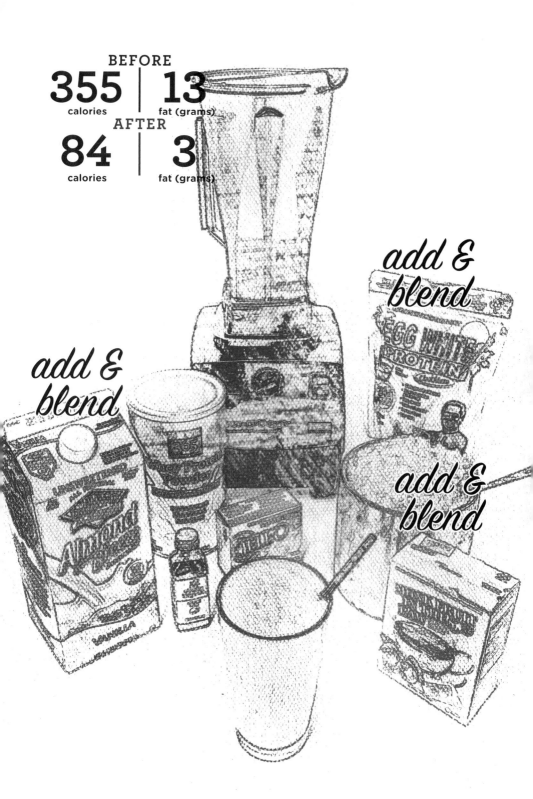

ALMOND MILK SMOOTHIE

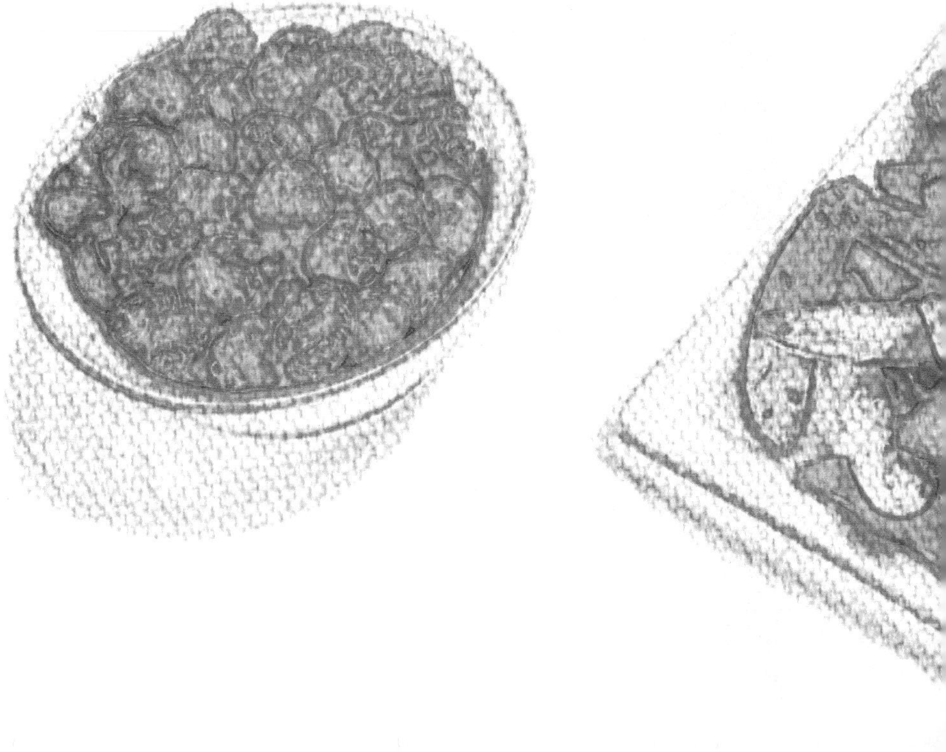

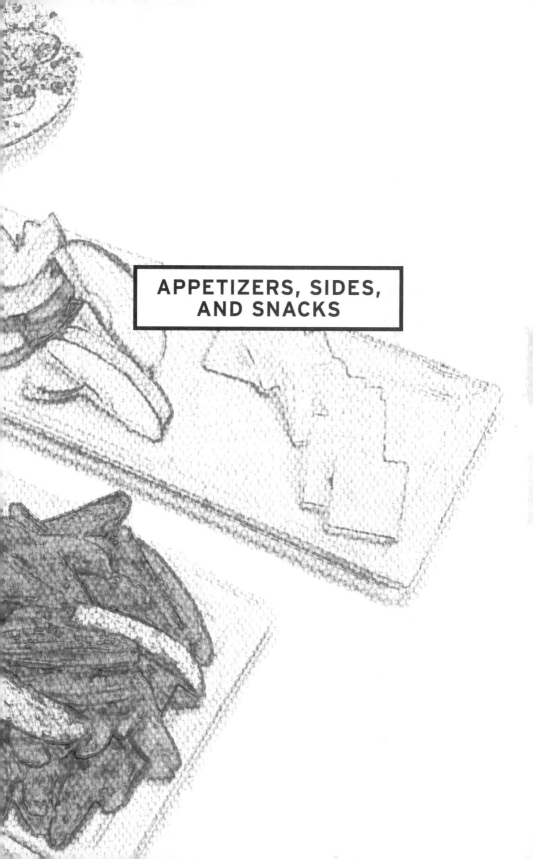

APPETIZERS, SIDES, AND SNACKS

FRESH WASABI PEAS

C | 29
F | 0g

WE ALL NEED great snacks, salty, crunchy snacks that will keep us happy between meals. I've taken a cue from a super-popular Japanese snack of dried peas coated with wasabi and made them healthy. Store-bought wasabi peas are a great snack as compared to chips, but you do need to read the label, as most have added fat, starches, and sugar. I use low-calorie-density sweet snap peas and add a zap of metabolism-boosting wasabi and sea salt to create a safely addictive snack that can be kept in the refrigerator for a few days for you to munch on. Plus, these are great to serve to friends with toothpicks for easy noshing.

Yield:	Prep time:	Cooking time:
4 snack or side dish servings	about 1 minute	3 minutes

Ingredients:

1   **teaspoon no-added-salt-or-sugar wasabi powder (such as Eden)**

4   **cups cleaned sugar snap peas (available in bags in the produce department)**
     Coarse sea salt (such as kosher), to taste

Method:

1. *Mix* the wasabi powder with 1 teaspoon of water in a large mixing bowl and let stand for 5 minutes.

2. *Bring* 2 quarts of water to a boil, add 1 teaspoon salt, and *submerge* the peas in the water. *Cook* the peas for 30 seconds, *drain* in a colander, and *shock* them in ice water to chill, about 1 minute. *Drain* the peas and *pat* dry with a clean towel.

3. *Add* the peas to the bowl with the wasabi, *toss* to coat, *season* with salt, and serve.

Tips:

- You can skip the cooking step altogether and eat these peas raw if they're tender and fresh enough.
- These peas make a great pairing with ANY grilled fish.

Per serving:

29 calories, 0g fat (0g sat), 0mg cholesterol, 65mg sodium, 5g carbohydrate, 1.8g fiber, 1.8g protein

Nutrient content claims:

Low calorie / Fat free / Saturated fat free / Cholesterol free / Low sodium / Trans fat free / Gluten free

> *Recommended ready-made version:*
> Hapi Snacks Hot Wasabi Peas
> Calories: 130 / Fat: 4g

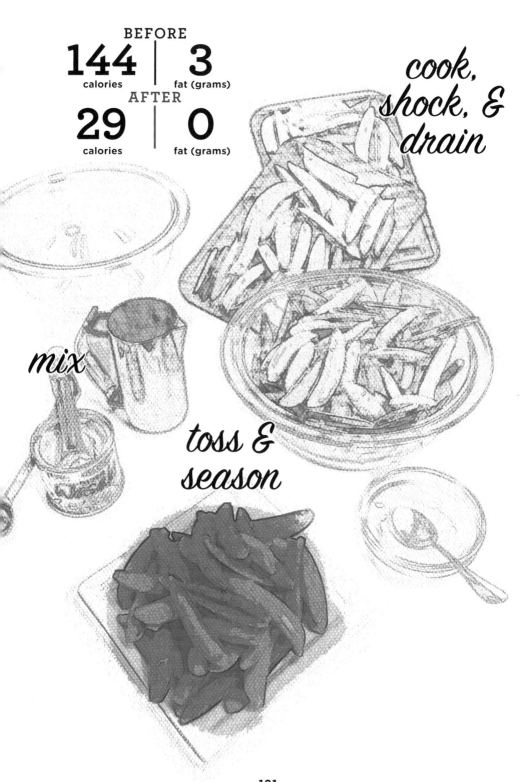

BEFORE

144 | **3**
calories | fat (grams)

AFTER

29 | **0**
calories | fat (grams)

*cook,
shock, &
drain*

mix

*toss &
season*

121

FRESH WASABI PEAS

SWEET POTATO CHIPS

C | 37
F | 0g

CRUNCHY, SALTY SNACKS are so easy to enjoy but just so bad for our bodies. Here I've eliminated the usual fat with a microwave technique and replaced the white potato with a much more nutritious sweet potato for this wonderful chip seasoned with one of my favorite seasoning mixes! These are a great alternative to fries with my RD's Big Burger with All the Fixin's.

Yield:	Prep time:	Cooking time:
4 servings	about 5 minutes	about 5 minutes

Ingredients:

Olive oil cooking spray (such as Pam)

½ **teaspoon Old Bay seasoning**

6 **ounces sweet potato, peeled and sliced ⅛ inch thick on a mandoline**

Method:

1. *Spray* a large microwave-safe plate with 1 second of cooking spray and *sprinkle* a little Old Bay seasoning on the bottom of the plate. *Place* some of the sweet potato slices on the plate in a *single layer. Spray* with 1 second of the cooking spray and then sprinkle each slice with some Old Bay. *Microwave* on high heat for 1 minute. *Flip* over each chip and microwave until the chips are lightly browned and crisp, about another minute.

2. Repeat the first step until all the remaining potato slices are cooked. Serve immediately or store in an airtight container for later use.

Tip:

- Try some other flavors and spices, like your favorite BBQ spice rub, or curry, or you can find some really fine flavors online, like sour cream and onion!

Per serving:

37 calories, 0g fat (0g sat), 0mg cholesterol, 103.5mg sodium, 8.5g carbohydrate, 1.5g fiber, 1g protein

Nutrient content claims:

Low calorie / Fat free / Saturated fat free / Trans fat free / Low sodium / Cholesterol free / Gluten free / No added sugar

> *Recommended ready-made version:*
> Rhythm Superfoods sweet potato chips
> Calories: 100 / Fat: 0g

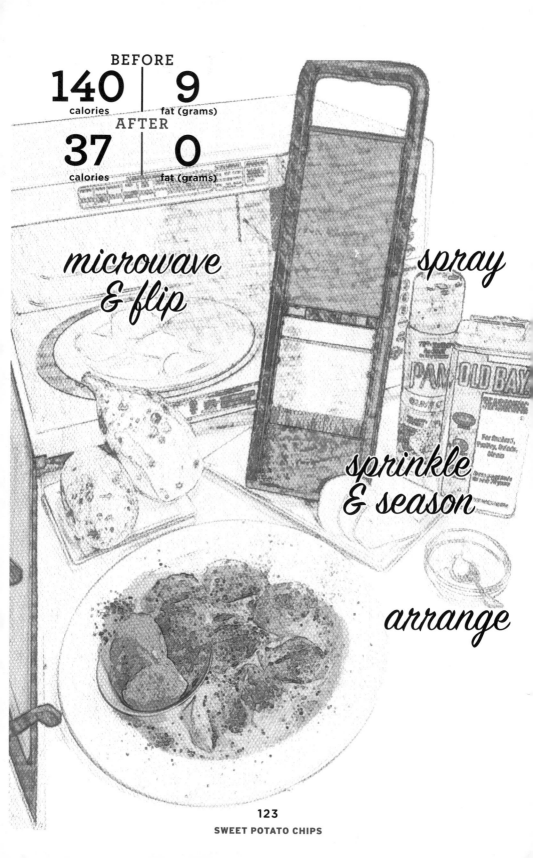

BEFORE

140 calories | **9** fat (grams)

AFTER

37 calories | **0** fat (grams)

microwave & flip

spray

sprinkle & season

arrange

CRISPY HOT AND SWEET GARBANZOS

C | 90
F | 1.5g

THIS GREAT HEALTHY snack will transport your taste buds to the Mediterranean with its flavors and will keep you on track with the philosophies of the Mediterranean diet. High in protein and using the fat found in the olives, this metabolism-boosting snack gets its zing from harissa powder.

Yield:	Prep time:	Cooking time:
4 servings	about 1 minute	3 to 5 minutes

Ingredients:

2   cups no-salt-added canned garbanzo beans (such as Kuner's)
2   teaspoons harissa powder (such as Kula!)
2   packets monk fruit extract (such as Monk Fruit In The Raw)
    Salt
    Olive oil cooking spray (such as Pam)

Method:

1. *Drain* the garbanzo beans and pat dry with a towel. *Place* the beans in a large mixing bowl, *dust* with the harissa powder, and *season* with the monk fruit extract and salt. *Spray* the beans with 3 seconds of cooking spray and *distribute* them on a microwave-safe plate.

2. Put the plate in the microwave and *cook* the beans on high until they're dried and crispy but not browned, 3 to 5 minutes. Remove from the microwave and let cool to room temperature. Serve.

Tip:

• Place the beans in a salad spinner, if you have one handy, to get as much water off them as possible.

Per serving:

90 calories, 1.5g fat (0g sat), 0mg cholesterol, 10mg sodium, 15g carbohydrate, 2g fiber, 5g protein

Nutrient content claims:

Reduced calorie / Low fat / Saturated fat free / Cholesterol free / Low sodium / No added sugar / Trans fat free / Gluten free

> *Recommended ready-made version:*
> SnackChicks Hot Chicks
> Calories: 120 / Fat: 3g

season & dust

drain

125

CRISPY HOT AND SWEET GARBANZOS

SUPER POPCORN-KALE CRUMBLE

C | 40
F | 0g

AIR-POPPED popcorn is a great snack, and when it's loaded with the nutrients of kale and the metabolism boost of crushed red pepper flakes, it becomes a Super Snack!

Yield:	Prep time:	Cooking time:
4 servings	about 2 minutes	about 3 minutes

Ingredients:

1   bunch Tuscan kale (about 18 leaves), leaves only
     Olive oil cooking spray (such as Pam)
4   cups air-popped popcorn
     Salt and crushed red pepper flakes

Method:

1. *Lay* the kale out on a microwave-safe plate, *spray* with 1 second of cooking spray, and *cook* on high for 1 minute. *Flip* the leaves and cook on high until the leaves are dried and crisp, about another minute.

2. *Toss* the kale crisps with the popcorn, *season* with salt and crushed red pepper flakes, and serve in a bowl.

Tip:

- Add some ripped nori paper for a nice flavor and a good boost of nutrition from the seaweed's high fiber, protein, and vitamin C content.

Per serving:

40 calories, 0g fat (0g sat), 0mg cholesterol, 8mg sodium, 8g carbohydrate, 1.5g fiber, 1.5g protein

Nutrient content claims:

Low calorie / Fat free / Saturated fat free / Cholesterol free / Low sodium / No added sugar / Trans fat free / Gluten free

Recommended ready-made version:
Orville Redenbacher's Light Natural Simply Salted 50% Less Fat microwave popcorn snack
Calories: 20 / Fat: 1g

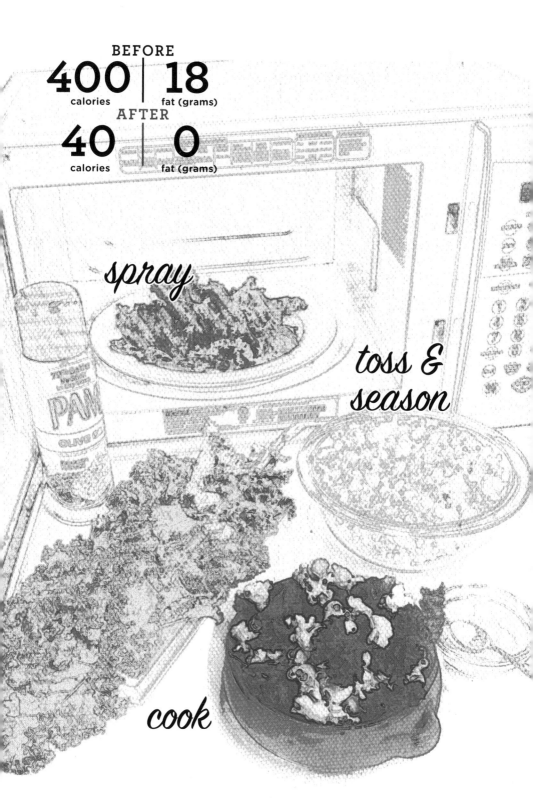

BEFORE

400 | **18**
calories | fat (grams)

AFTER

40 | **0**
calories | fat (grams)

spray

toss &
season

cook

APPLES AND CHEDDAR CHEESE

C | 117
F | 2.5g

A SUPER-QUICK on-the-go snack option.

| Yield: | Prep time: |
| 4 servings | about 2 minutes |

Ingredients:

4   cups sliced apples

4   ounces 75% reduced-fat cheddar cheese (such as Cabot)

Method:

1. *Place* 1 cup of the apples on each plate. *Slice* the cheddar cheese into ¼-inch slices, *arrange* the cheese on each plate next to the apples, and serve.

Tip:

- I like Pink Lady apples, Gala apples, and Winesaps.

Per serving:

117 calories, 2.5g fat (1.525g sat), 10mg cholesterol, 201mg sodium, 15.5g carbohydrate, 2.5g fiber, 9.25g protein

Nutrient content claims:

Reduced calorie / Low fat / Low cholesterol / No added sugar / Good source of fiber / Trans fat free / Gluten free

---

Recommended ready-made version:
WonderSlim Cheddar Crunchers
Calories: 130 / Fat: 5g

BEFORE
282 | **15.5**
calories | fat (grams)
AFTER
117 | **2.5**
calories | fat (grams)

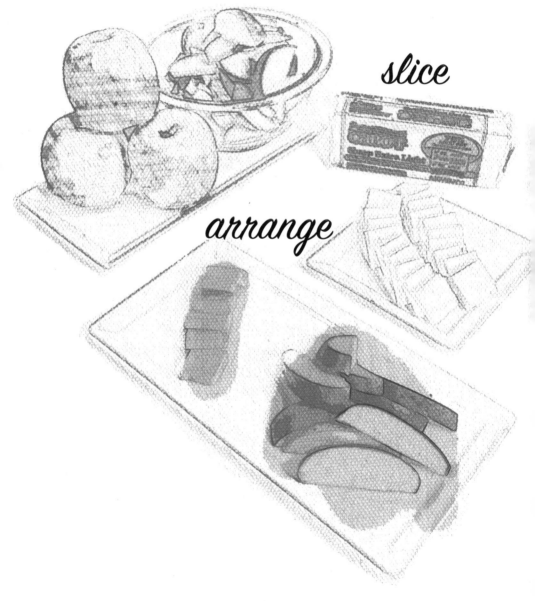

slice

arrange

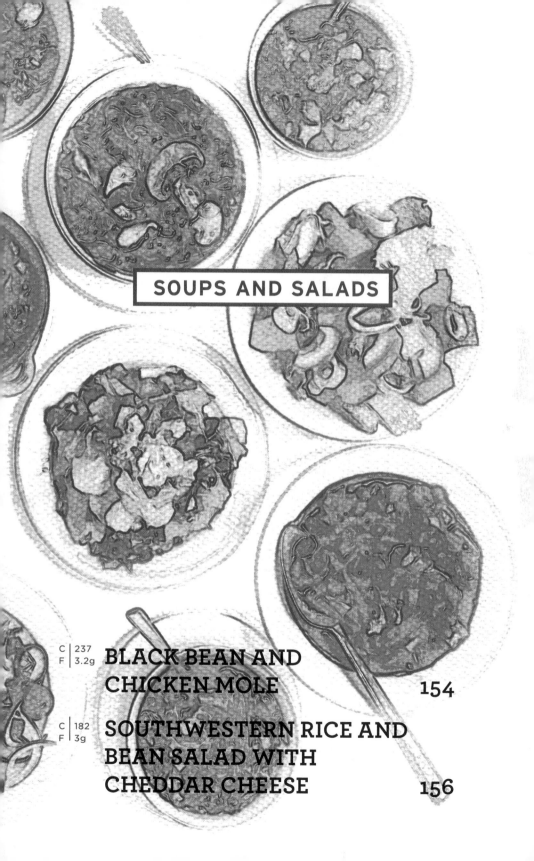

SOUPS AND SALADS

MUSHROOM MISO
NOODLE SOUP

C | 49
F | 0g

FALL is a great time for a robust mushroom soup. Cream of mushroom soups are the standby, but besides being less healthy, sometimes all that dairy gets in the way of the subtle flavors of the fresh mushrooms. This simple soup has a deceivingly and surprisingly complex flavor. By using miso, I can build a very good base for a soup in seconds that works well with the earthy, low-calorie-density mushrooms. By adding some leafy greens, I add even more nutrients to this already healthy soup. This allows us to enjoy more of that wonderful mushroom flavor and stay healthy and feeling good.

Yield:	Prep time:	Cooking time:
4 servings	about 2 minutes	about 5 minutes

Ingredients:

16   ounces shirataki noodles, rinsed well and drained

1   quart fat-free, reduced-sodium chicken broth (such as Swanson's)

1¹/₂   tablespoons miso paste

10   ounces mixed mushrooms, cut into bite-sized pieces

4   cups tightly packed spinach leaves

Salt and freshly ground black pepper

Method:

1. *Put* the noodles in a 4-quart saucepot and set over medium-high heat. Stir and *cook* until all the residual water is evaporated and the noodles are hot, about 30 seconds. *Add* the broth, miso, and mushrooms, cover, and bring to a *simmer*.

2. Remove the lid, *add* the spinach leaves, and stir them in to *wilt*. *Season* with salt and pepper if needed. Divide the soup among four bowls and serve.

Tips:

- White, or shiro, miso is the most widely available in supermarkets. If you can find other varieties of miso, experiment to find out which one—or which combination—you like the best! Try half-and-half white and red, or aka, miso if you can find it.
- This is a great soup base that you can add to. Try grated ginger for some zing, or try thinly sliced snow peas or spinach for added fiber, or even add some shrimp, diced tofu, or fish for added protein and still be under 100 calories.

Per serving:

49 calories, 0g fat (0g sat), 0mg cholesterol, 298.75mg sodium, 6.5g carbohydrate, 1.5g fiber, 6g protein

Nutrient content claims:

Reduced calorie / Fat free / Saturated fat free / Cholesterol free / No added sugar / Trans fat free / Gluten free

Recommended ready-made version:
Amy's No Chicken Noodle Soup
Calories: 90 / Fat: 3g

BEFORE

311
calories

8
fat (grams)

AFTER

49
calories

0
fat (grams)

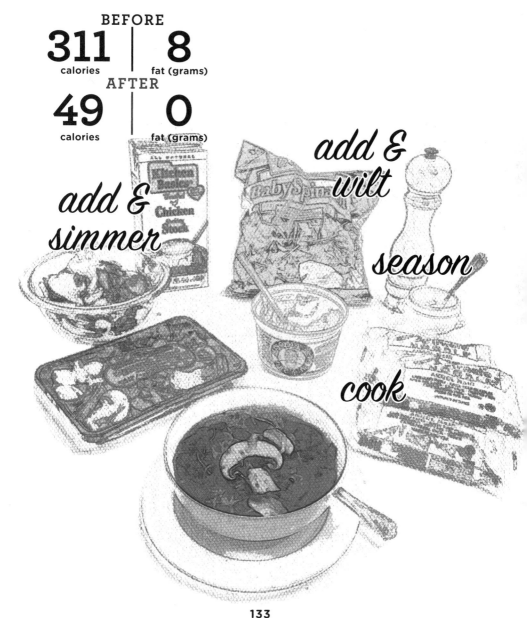

*add &
simmer*

*add &
wilt*

season

cook

MUSHROOM MISO NOODLE SOUP

MEDITERRANEAN TUNA SALAD

C | 90
F | 1g

I LOVE THIS tuna chopped salad, super-quick and super-delicious. I like keeping my body "up" during the day with low-calorie-density vegetables that keep the metabolism working and leave me feeling energetic and sharp. I eliminate oil here by relying on the texture of the capers, along with the seeds and skins of the cherry tomatoes, to hold on to the vegetables' nooks and crannies. This will change the way you think about tuna salad!

Yield:	Prep time:
4 servings	about 5 minutes

Ingredients:

1   pint cherry tomatoes, cut in half

4   tablespoons capers, drained and chopped

3   cups fresh chopped vegetable medley (such as Ready Pac Salad Confetti)

1   head butter lettuce, torn into 1-inch pieces

    Salt and freshly ground black pepper

8   ounces water-packed no-added-salt light tuna, drained (such as Sustainable Seas)

Method:

1. *Combine* the tomatoes and capers in a blender or food processor and *process* on low until you have a watery yet chunky dressing that will adhere to the salad.

2. *Place* the vegetables and lettuce in a bowl, add the dressing, *season* with salt and pepper, and *toss* to coat everything evenly.

3. Spoon the mixture evenly onto four plates and *top* each salad with 2 ounces of tuna.

Tips:

- Look for vegetable mixes that include cauliflower, cabbage, broccoli, zucchini, and carrots.
- Add ¼ cup basil to lift up the freshness for an additional 2 calories per serving.
- Try adding 1 teaspoon of prepared horseradish to the tomato and caper dressing for a delicious metabolism booster with only an added 2 calories!

Per serving:

90 calories, 1g fat (0g sat), 25mg cholesterol, 380.75mg sodium, 8g carbohydrate, 3g fiber, 3g protein

Reduced calorie / Low fat / Saturated fat free / No added sugar / Good source
of fiber / Trans fat free / Gluten free

Recommended ready-made version:
Starkist Tuna Salad Sandwich
Calories: 100 / Fat: 3.5g

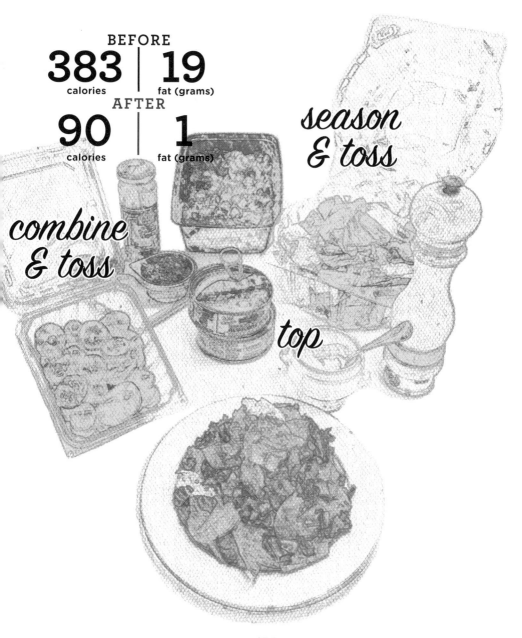

BEFORE
383 | **19**
calories | fat (grams)

AFTER
90 | **1**
calories | fat (grams)

season & toss

combine & toss

top

TURKEY AND LENTIL SOUP

C | 204
F | 1g

LENTILS ARE SOME of the healthiest little legumes on the earth. They're great for endless reasons: not only are they low in fat and calories and high in fiber and protein, but they also contain high levels of flavonols, which at least one study has found to lower the risk of breast cancer! Lentils unfortunately take an hour to cook, but there are some great all-natural cooked products out there, so this soup can be made in less than 5 minutes, and you don't even need to pick up a knife!

Yield:	Prep time:	Cooking time:
4 servings	about 1 minute	about 4 minutes

Ingredients:

Olive oil cooking spray (such as Pam)

2   cups precut fresh mirepoix (diced onion, carrot, celery—look in the produce department)

½   tablespoon sweet smoked paprika

2   cups ready-to-eat cooked lentils (such as Melissa's or Eden)

6   ounces reduced-sodium smoked turkey breast, shredded into small pieces (such as Boar's Head)

1   quart plus 1 cup fat-free reduced-sodium chicken broth (such as Swanson's)
     Salt and freshly ground black pepper

Method:

1. *Spray* a wide 4-quart saucepot with cooking spray, place over medium-high heat, add the mirepoix and paprika, and *cook*, covered, stirring occasionally, until it begins to steam, about 30 seconds. *Add* the lentils, turkey, and broth, *cover*, and bring to a *simmer*.

2. Remove the lid, *season* with salt (if needed) and pepper, and serve.

Tips:

• Finish each serving of soup with a few grinds of black pepper—this is just the kind of dish that cries for it!

• If you're a fan of a heartier soup, blend one-third of the soup in a blender once the stock is added, then put it back in the pot.

• I love smoky flavors with lentils, but for a switch, try using curry powder instead of the paprika.

Per serving:

204 calories, 1g fat (0g sat), 18.75mg cholesterol, 705.5mg sodium, 25.5g carbohydrate, 9.5g fiber, 23.75g protein

Nutrient content claims:

Low fat / Saturated fat free / Low cholesterol / No added sugar / High fiber / High protein / Trans fat free / Gluten free

BEFORE

260 | **12**
calories | fat (grams)

AFTER

204 | **1**
calories | fat (grams)

spray

cook

add, cover, & simmer

season

TOMATO AND SHRIMP KIMCHI SALAD

C | 116
F | 1g

I LOVE CAPRESE SALAD—it's built into my heritage and upbringing, after all—but wouldn't it be nice to have an alternative up your sleeve, and an even healthier one to boot? Here it is, the sweetness of tomatoes paired with the probiotic cruciferous cabbage condiment from Korea called kimchi. The metabolism-boosting Korean chili pepper is refreshed by the fresh herbs and low-calorie-density tomatoes, giving this dish such a round, bold flavor you'll never miss those oil- or mayo-laden shrimp salads.

Yield:	Prep time:	Cooking time:
4 servings	about 2 minutes	about 2 minutes

Ingredients:

2   cups broccoli slaw (such as Dole)
1/2   cup spicy-as-you-can-handle kimchi, roughly chopped, plus 1/4 cup liquid
2   pints cherry tomatoes, cut in half
    Salt and freshly ground black pepper
8   ounces cooked domestic shrimp
1/2   cup cilantro, picked off the largest stem, cut into 2-inch pieces

Method:

1. *Combine* the broccoli slaw, kimchi, and liquid in a large mixing bowl and add the cherry tomatoes. *Stir* to combine and season with salt and pepper to taste. *Add* the shrimp, *toss* to coat everything, then divide the mixture among four shallow serving bowls. *Top* each bowl evenly with the cilantro and serve.

Tips:

• Use the ripest tomatoes you can find; the variety doesn't really matter.
• Feel free to add mint and/or basil to give this a super-fresh lift without adding calories.

Per serving:

116 calories, 1g fat (0g sat), 110.75mg cholesterol, 508.25mg sodium, 12.4g carbohydrate, 3.4g fiber, 14.2g protein

Nutrient content claims:

Reduced calorie / Reduced fat / Low fat / Saturated fat free / Good source of fiber / High protein / Trans fat free / Gluten free

> *Recommended ready-made version:*
> Supermarket salad bar cucumber tomato salad
> Calories: 140 / Fat: 0g

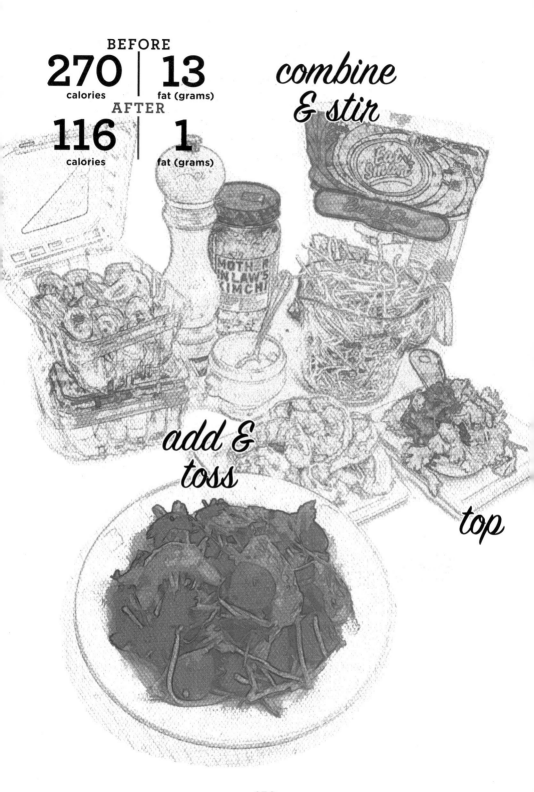

270 calories | 13 fat (grams)

116 calories | 1 fat (grams)

combine & stir

add & toss

top

TOMATO AND SHRIMP KIMCHI SALAD

TOMATO AND VEGETABLE SOUP

C | 74
F | 0g

THIS QUICK SOUP can be made with detoxifying cruciferous vegetables, like the cauliflower and broccoli found in frozen vegetable medleys. You can make this entirely in the microwave by adding the broth and V8 to the bowl after the vegetables are cooked, but it's a little precarious to handle that amount of very hot liquid with such viscosity in a bowl.

Yield:	Prep time:	Cooking time:
4 servings	about 2 minutes	about 5 minutes

Ingredients:

2	cups low-sodium V8
2	cups fat-free, reduced-sodium chicken broth (such as Swanson's)
12	ounces drained and rinsed shirataki noodles (such as Miracle Noodle Angel Hair)
3	cups fresh frozen vegetable mix (such as Birds Eye Steamfresh)
	Salt and freshly ground black pepper
¼	cup fresh basil leaves, torn into bite-sized pieces

Method:

1. In a medium saucepot, *heat* the V8, chicken broth, and noodles to a *simmer*, about 5 minutes. Place the vegetables in any type of food processor and *pulse* to chop them into small pieces, but not pureed.

2. *Place* the vegetables in a microwave-safe bowl, cover with plastic wrap, and *cook* on high until the vegetables are tender, about 2 minutes.

3. Add the cooked vegetables to the saucepot, *season* with salt and pepper, and *add* the basil. Ladle the soup into four bowls and serve.

Tips:

- Add trimmed and broiled beef tenderloin chunks for an additional 2 grams of fat and 50 calories per ounce—beef and noodle soup for 124 calories!
- Add some crushed red pepper flakes for a spicy soup to get that metabolism boosted for 0 calories.

Per serving:
74 calories, 0g fat (0g sat), 0mg cholesterol, 154.7mg sodium, 12.4g carbohydrate, 3g fiber, 3.8g protein

Nutrient content claims:
Reduced calorie / Fat free / Saturated fat free / Cholesterol free / No added sugar / Good source of fiber / Trans fat free / Gluten free

BEFORE

284 | 8
calories | fat (grams)

AFTER

74 | 0
calories | fat (grams)

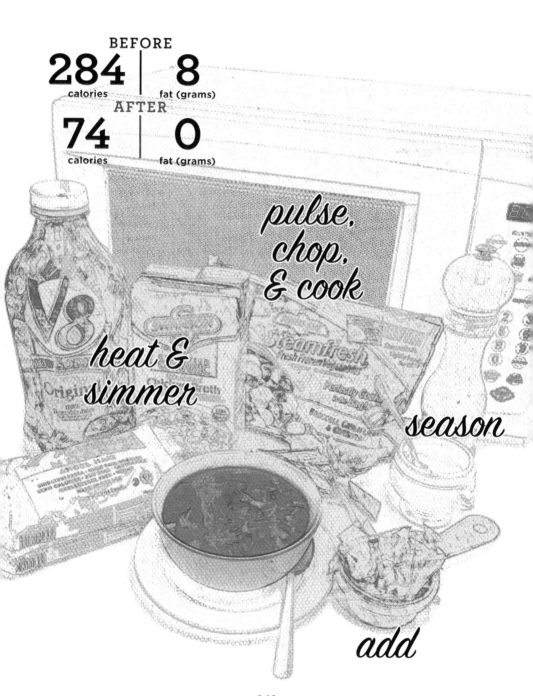

pulse, chop, & cook

heat & simmer

season

add

141

OLD-FASHIONED CHICKEN NOODLE SOUP

C | 191
F | 3g

CHICKEN NOODLE SOUP has long been lauded as soup for the soul. However, some versions of it are not as good for your body as you might think. My recipe uses shirataki noodles, which have zero net carbs, zero calories, and zero gluten. This recipe also yields almost 24 ounces per portion, which is three times that of a normal soup, so you can fill up for just under 200 calories! Packed with low-calorie-density vegetables and a low-sodium, fat-free chicken broth, my chicken noodle soup not only can cure a somber soul but can actually keep you healthy and trim. Also, these noodles will never overcook, so you can make this soup and keep it for days without having soggy noodles!

This is a great base recipe for noodle soup. You can add different herbs and spices to take it in any direction. Some soy, ginger, and bok choy; or miso and mushrooms; or even some kimchi and peas are great ways to keep it interesting while not abandoning the core goal of cooking delicious food that's good for you.

Yield:	Prep time:	Cooking time:
4 servings	about 1 minute	about 5 minutes

Ingredients:

8   cups reduced-sodium, fat-free chicken broth (such as Swanson's)
1/2   cube salt-free vegetable bouillon (such as Rapunzel)
10   ounces skinless, boneless store-roasted chicken, shredded
16   ounces shirataki noodles, rinsed in cold water and drained
4   cups precut fresh mirepoix (diced onion, carrot, celery—look in the produce department)
     Old Bay seasoning
     Freshly ground black pepper

Method:

1. Place the chicken broth in a wide saucepot with the bouillon cube, chicken, and noodles; *cover* and bring to a *simmer*. Place the vegetables in a microwave-safe bowl and *cook* on high until soft, 2 to 4 minutes.

2. Add the vegetables to the soup, *season* with Old Bay and pepper, and pour into four large soup bowls.

Tip:

• The yield given here is based on a quick boil. If the soup boils too long, there will be increased evaporation and the yield will be less.

Per serving:
191 calories, 3g fat (1g sat), 63mg cholesterol, 457mg sodium, 14g carbohydrate, 2.4g fiber, 26g protein

Nutrient content claims:
Reduced calorie / Reduced fat / Low saturated fat / No added sugar / High protein / Trans fat free / Gluten free

Recommended ready-made version:
Progresso Light Chicken Noodle Soup (8 ounces)
Calories: 70 / Fat: 1.5g

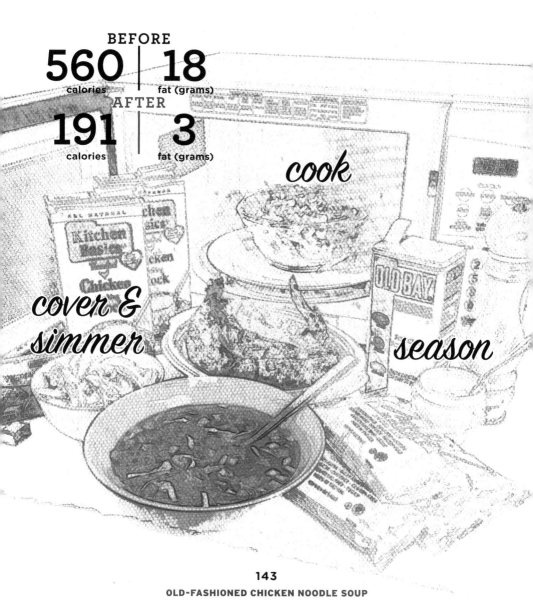

BEFORE
560 | **18**
calories | fat (grams)

AFTER
191 | **3**
calories | fat (grams)

cook

cover & simmer

season

CALAMARI AND WATERMELON SALAD

C | 167
F | 6g

A GREAT, refreshing salad composed in a flash.

Yield:	Prep time:	Cooking time:
4 servings	about 1 minute	about 4 minutes

Ingredients:

4   hot pickled cherry peppers, chopped, plus 4 tablespoons pepper liquid
4   cups store-prepared, no-sugar-added diced watermelon
1   avocado, peeled and diced into bite-sized pieces
4   cups store-chopped hearts of romaine
    Olive oil cooking spray (such as Pam)
8   ounces cleaned calamari, cut into rings (your fishmonger can do this for you)
    Salt and freshly ground pepper

Method:

1. Put the peppers and their liquid, the watermelon, and the avocado in a large bowl and gently *toss* to coat. *Add* the romaine, *toss* gently again to coat, and divide among four salad bowls.

2. *Spray* a large nonstick skillet with cooking spray and place over high heat. *Season* the calamari with salt and pepper. Once the skillet is hot, add the calamari and *cook* until browned and cooked through, about 1 minute. Evenly distribute the cooked calamari over each salad and serve.

Per serving:

167 calories, 6g fat (0.9g sat), 131.75mg cholesterol, 187mg sodium, 18.6g carbohydrate, 3.9g fiber, 10.9g protein

Nutrient content claims:

Reduced calorie / Low saturated fat / Good source of fiber / High protein / Trans fat free / Gluten free

Recommended ready-made version:
Supermarket salad bar watermelon and lettuce
Calories: 45 / Fat: 0g

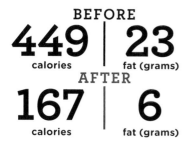

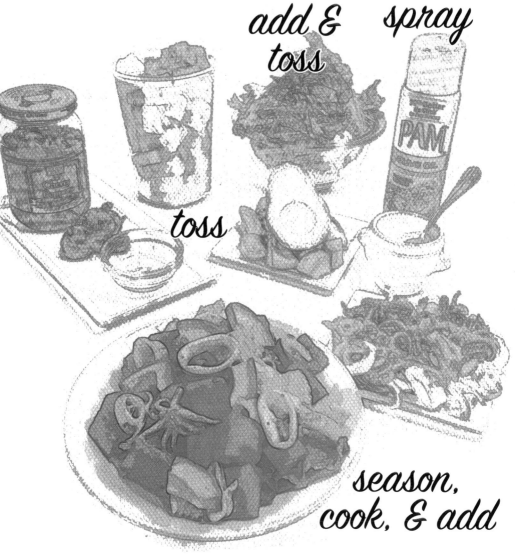

*add &
toss*

spray

toss

*season,
cook, & add*

SALMON AND CUCUMBER SALAD WITH CREAMY DILL DRESSING

C | 171
F | 4g

THE CLASSIC FLAVORS of salmon, cream, and dill come together here in a very filling and reduced-fat salad that can be prepared quickly.

Yield:	Prep time:	Cooking time:
4 servings	about 1 minute	about 2 minutes

Ingredients:

- ½ cup fat-free Greek yogurt (such as Fage Total 0%)
- 3 tablespoons fresh lemon juice
- ¼ cup fresh dill, chopped
- 6 cups store-prepared plain cucumber, onion, and cherry tomato salad (find it in the salad bar section or deli counter at the supermarket)
  Salt and cayenne pepper
- 8 ounces canned no-added-salt sockeye salmon, drained

Method:

1. *Mix* the yogurt, lemon juice, and dill in a large mixing bowl until smooth. *Add* the cucumber salad, *toss* to coat the vegetables evenly, and *season* with salt and cayenne pepper to taste.

2. Divide the salad among four plates and *top* each with an equal amount of salmon.

Tip:

- Try using green or red hot sauce in place of the cayenne pepper for a little added zing.

Per serving:

171 calories, 4g fat (1 g sat), 25mg cholesterol, 104mg sodium, 17.5g carbohydrate, 1.5g fiber, 16g protein

Nutrient content claims:

Reduced calories / Reduced fat / Low saturated fat / No added sugar / Low sodium / Trans fat free / Gluten free / High protein

> *Recommended ready-made version:*
> Lean Cuisine Salmon with Basil
> Calories: 210 / Fat: 6g

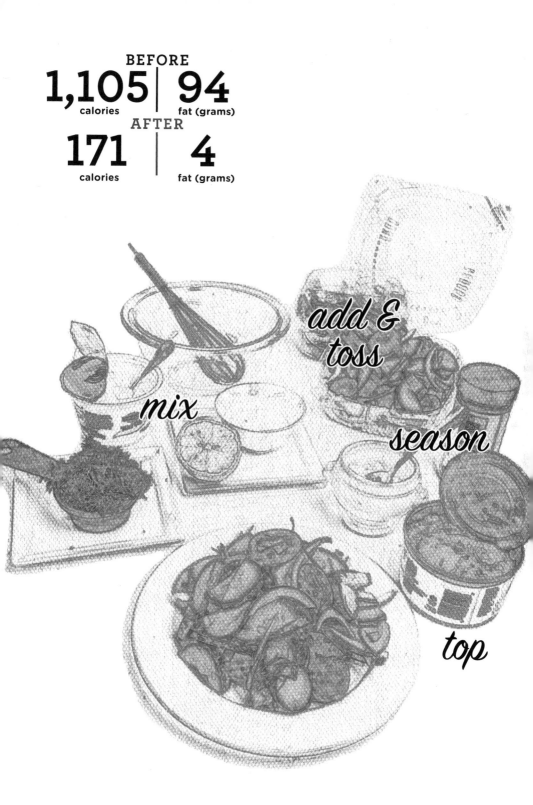

mix

add & toss

season

top

SALMON AND CUCUMBER SALAD WITH CREAMY DILL DRESSING

CRUNCHY KALE, APPLE, AND POMEGRANATE SALAD

C | 126
F | 4.5g

RAW KALE is high-octane food as far as your body is concerned, and this recipe will have your taste buds craving it as well. This salad gets a boost from ingredients that are naturally sweet and sour, the pumpkin seeds have good fat, and the salad dresses itself!

Yield:	Prep time:	Processing time:
4 servings	about 2 minutes	about 2 minutes

Ingredients:

3   tablespoons shelled unsalted pumpkin seeds
3   tablespoons red wine vinegar
1/4 cup fat-free Greek yogurt (such as Fage Total 0%)
6   cups Tuscan kale, washed and chopped into 1-inch pieces (the supermarket sells this ready to use!)
1   cup Granny Smith apple, diced into bite-sized pieces
1/2 cup pomegranate seeds (such as POM Wonderful)
     Salt and crushed red pepper flakes

Method:

1. Place the pumpkin seeds on a microwave-safe plate and *cook* on high until they're golden brown, about 2 minutes. Reserve.

2. Place the vinegar and yogurt in a large mixing bowl and *stir* together. Put the kale, apple, and pomegranate seeds in a large bowl, *toss* together, and add the pumpkin seeds. *Season* with salt and crushed red pepper flakes and serve.

Per serving:

126 calories, 4.5g fat (2.9g sat), 0mg cholesterol, 49.25mg sodium, 17.7g carbohydrate, 2.1g fiber, 9g protein

Nutrient content claims:

Reduced calorie / Reduced fat / Cholesterol free / Low sodium / No added sugar / Trans fat free / Gluten free

> *Recommended ready-made version:*
> Whole Foods Prepared Kale Salad with Chili Lime Dressing
> Calories: 130 / Fat: 6g

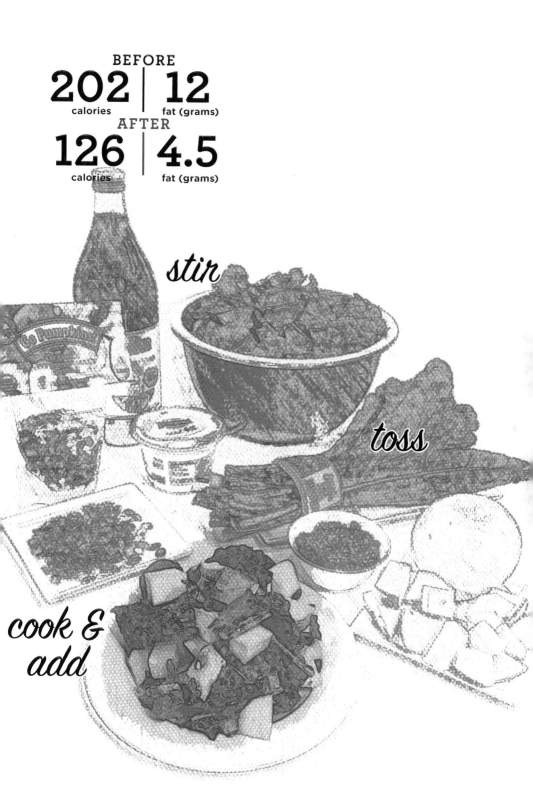

BEFORE

202 | **12**
calories | fat (grams)

AFTER

126 | **4.5**
calories | fat (grams)

stir

toss

*cook &
add*

CRUNCHY KALE, APPLE, AND POMEGRANATE SALAD

GRILLED SHRIMP GAZPACHO

C | 140
F | 1g

GAZPACHO, as it was originated in southern Spain, is made by finely cutting fresh vegetables, adding them to fresh tomato puree, and thickening it with pureed bread! Naturally, I eliminated the bread (and the knife work!) and added a protein punch from shrimp. I came up with this soup so vivid with fresh flavors you'd think it took an hour to make.

Yield:	Prep time:	Cooking time:
4 servings	about 1 minute	about 4 minutes

Ingredients:

1   pint spicy store-bought pico de gallo (such as Ready Pac)

1   pint mild store-bought pico de gallo (such as Ready Pac)

2   cups fresh-cut, store-bought vegetable mix (broccoli, cauliflower, peppers, etc.)
    Salt and freshly ground black pepper

12 ounces store-prepared boiled shrimp, shells removed

1   cup fresh cilantro sprigs, torn into bite-sized pieces

4   lime wedges for serving

Method:

1. Preheat a grill, grill pan, or nonstick pan over medium-high heat.

2. Pour the two pico de gallos into a blender and *blend* until smooth, about 30 seconds. Add the vegetable mix and *pulse* until well chopped. *Season* with salt and pepper, stir, and pour the gazpacho into four cold soup bowls.

3. *Season* the shrimp with salt and pepper and cook on the *grill* or pan until warmed through, about 1 minute per side. Distribute the shrimp evenly over the gazpacho, then *top* with the cilantro. Serve each bowl with a fresh lime wedge.

Tips:

• You can add a little water to the gazpacho if it's too thick for your taste.
• Try using Old Bay seasoning in place of the salt to season your shrimp!

Per serving:

140 calories, 1g fat (0g sat), 165.75mg cholesterol, 331.25mg sodium, 19g carbohydrate, 1g fiber, 18.9g protein

Nutrient content claims:

Reduced calorie / Low fat / Saturated fat free / No added sugar / High protein / Trans fat free / Gluten free

> *Recommended ready-made version:*
> Wegmans Gazpacho
> Calories: 80 / Fat: 4.55g

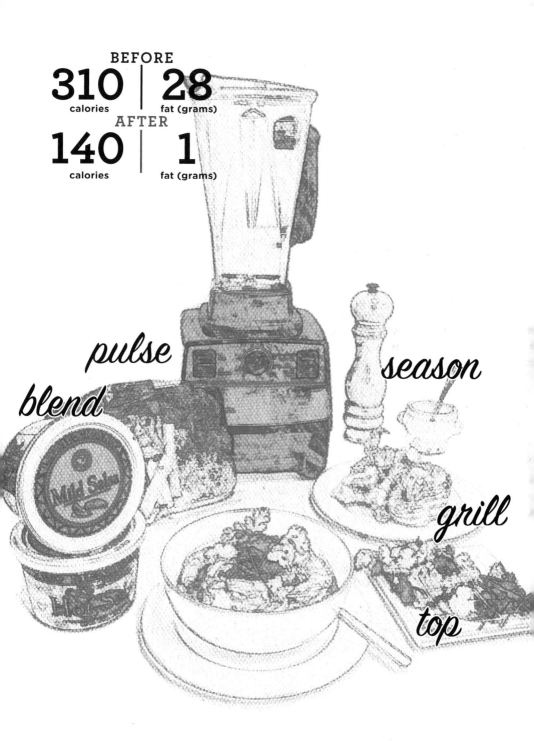

BEFORE

310 | **28**
calories | fat (grams)

AFTER

140 | **1**
calories | fat (grams)

pulse

blend

season

grill

top

MANHATTAN CLAM CHOWDER

C | 122
F | 1g

I GREW UP eating this soul-satisfying soup in a diner near my home. Diners of course are not known for their attention to calorie reduction, but as it turns out, this soup can be made even more delicious by removing all added fat. By eliminating the usual bacon and oil, the fresh oceanic flavor of the iron-rich clams really comes through and is nicely balanced by the fresh acidity of the lycopene-rich tomatoes.

Yield:	Prep time:	Cooking time:
4 servings	about 1 minute	about 4 minutes

Ingredients:

Olive oil cooking spray (such as Pam)

2   cups fresh diced tricolor peppers (such as Ready Pac, or you can use frozen)

2   cups fresh diced onions and celery (such as Ready Pac)

4   dozen littleneck clams with their juice, shucked and chopped by your fishmonger (call ahead so the clams are ready when you arrive!)

1½ cups no-added-sugar-or-salt chopped tomatoes (such as Pomi)

1½ tablespoons garlic flakes (such as Frontier)

Salt and freshly ground black pepper

Method:

1. *Spray* a large, wide saucepot with cooking spray, place over high heat, and *add* the peppers, onions, and celery. *Cook* until softened, about 2 minutes, then *add* the clams, clam juice, tomatoes, and garlic flakes.

2. Bring to a *simmer* and cook for 1 minute, season with salt and pepper, and divide among four large soup bowls.

Per serving:

122 calories, 1g fat (0g sat), 36.75mg cholesterol, 85.5mg sodium, 11g carbohydrate, 3.25g fiber, 15.5g protein

Nutrient content claims:

Reduced calorie / Low fat / Saturated fat free / Low sodium / No added sugar / Good source of fiber / High protein / Trans fat free / Gluten free

> *Recommended ready-made version:*
> Progresso Traditional Manhattan Clam Chowder
> Calories: 100 / Fat: 2g

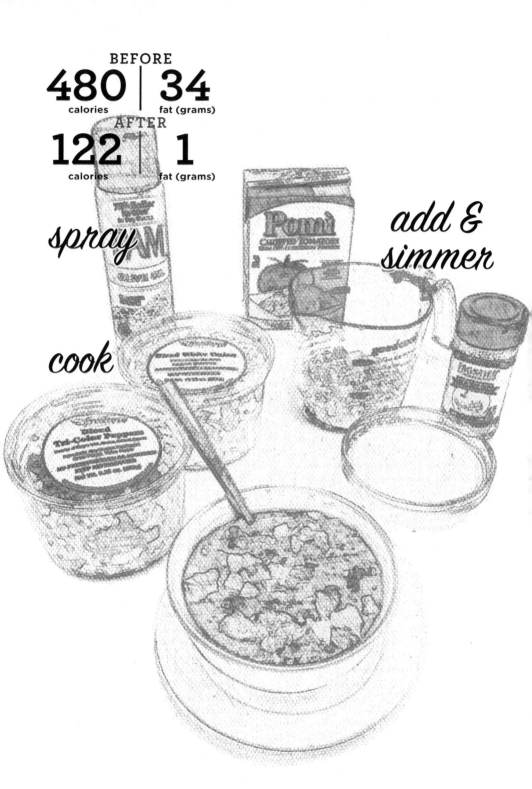

BEFORE

480 | **34**
calories | fat (grams)

AFTER

122 | **1**
calories | fat (grams)

spray

add & simmer

cook

BLACK BEAN AND CHICKEN MOLE

C | 237
F | 3g

TRAVEL SOUTH of the border with this deep and complex soup without even picking up a knife!

Yield:	Prep time:	Cooking time:
4 servings	about 1 minute	about 4 minutes

Ingredients:

1 quart reduced-sodium, fat-free chicken broth (such as Swanson's)

2 tablespoons salt-free mole spice (or substitute 1 tablespoon smoked paprika mixed with 1 tablespoon unsweetened cocoa powder, such as Hershey's Special Dark)

2 cups no-salt-added black beans (such as Eden), drained

8 ounces store-bought roasted chicken, skin removed, shredded

2 cups frozen pepper and onion mix (such as Birds Eye Pepper and Onion Stir-Fry)

Salt and freshly ground black pepper

4 lime wedges for serving

Method:

1. Put the broth and the spice mixture in a saucepot and *whisk* until all the spices are fully incorporated. *Add* the beans, chicken, and vegetables and bring to a *simmer*; *season* with salt and pepper.

2. Ladle the soup evenly into four bowls and serve each with a lime wedge.

Per serving:

237 calories, 3.2g fat (.5g sat), 50.5mg cholesterol, 290.75mg sodium, 24.5g carbohydrate, 9g fiber, 25g protein

Nutrient content claims:

Reduced calorie / Reduced fat / Low saturated fat / High fiber / High protein / No added sugar / Trans fat free / Gluten free

> *Recommended ready-made version:*
> Lean Cuisine Santa Fe–Style Rice and Beans
> Calories: 290 / Fat: 5g

BEFORE

524 | **18**
calories | fat (grams)

AFTER

237 | **3**
calories | fat (grams)

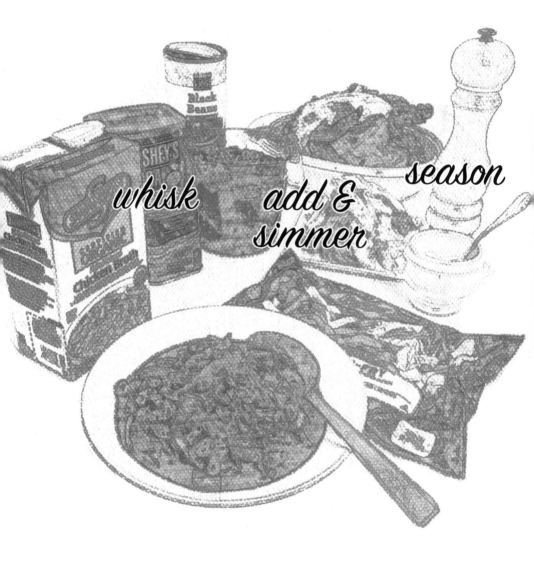

whisk

add & simmer

season

SOUTHWESTERN RICE AND BEAN SALAD WITH CHEDDAR CHEESE

C | 182
F | 3g

THIS POPULAR DISH is usually found in a wrap or burrito, which adds empty calories and fat. I make it as a rice bowl salad. Using a precooked brown-and-wild-rice blend with added vegetables and reduced-sodium cooked black beans, this high-flavored dish can be put together in minutes. I opted out of using corn and peppers in favor of a lower-calorie-density and higher-fiber iceberg salad, and it gives a nice fresh accent to the hot and filling rice, beans, and melted cheese.

Yield:	Prep time:
4 servings	about 2 minutes

Ingredients:

2   cups frozen brown and wild rice with vegetables (such as Birds Eye Steamfresh), defrosted
1   cup reduced-sodium black beans (such as Bush's)
    Salt-and-sodium-free adobo powder
1   cup prepared pico de gallo
5   cups iceberg lettuce, chopped
4   ounces 75% reduced-fat cheddar cheese (such as Cabot)

Method:

1. In a large bowl, *mix everything* together. *Season* with salt and pepper. Evenly divide among four bowls. No cooking, just toss and *serve.*

Tips:

- Add 1 ounce of cooked shrimp to each serving to get a protein and flavor boost for under 30 calories per portion!
- Use a microwave-safe plate to cover a bowl in the microwave and stack another bowl on top to save space and therefore time.

Per serving:

182 calories, 3g fat (1.5g sat), 10mg cholesterol, 317.25mg sodium, 28.4g carbohydrate, 5g fiber, 14.5g protein

Nutrient content claims:

Reduced calorie / Reduced fat / Low cholesterol / No added sugar / High fiber / High protein / Trans fat free / Gluten free

---

Recommended ready-made version:
Weight Watchers Smart Ones Santa Fe Style Rice & Beans
Calories: 310 / Fat: 7g

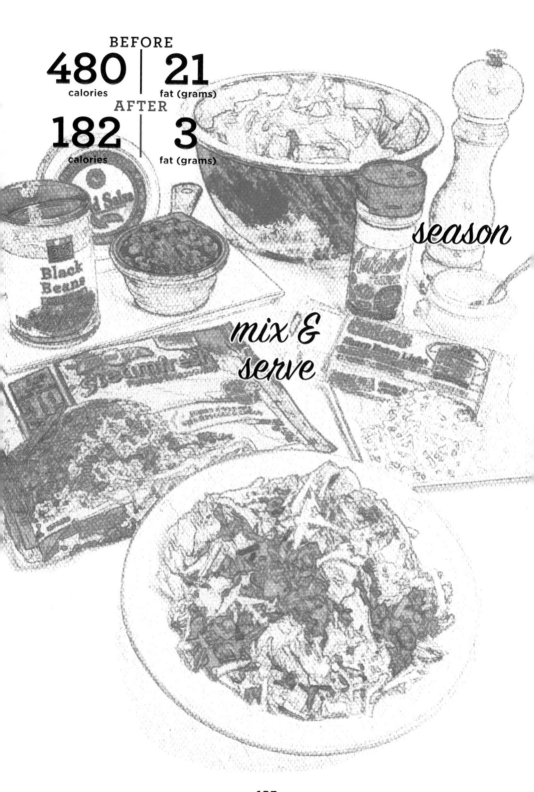

BEFORE

480 | **21**
calories | fat (grams)

AFTER

182 | **3**
calories | fat (grams)

season

*mix &
serve*

SOUTHWESTERN RICE AND BEAN SALAD WITH CHEDDAR CHEESE

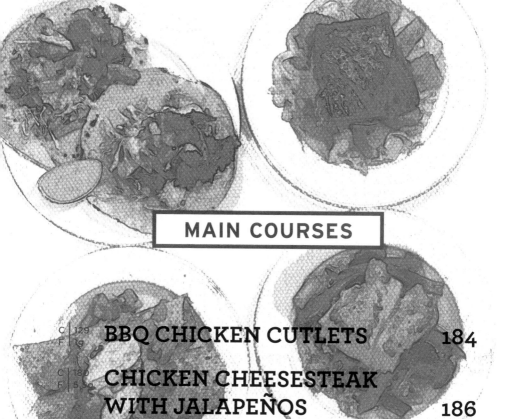

MAIN COURSES

ROTISSERIE CHICKEN AND TERIYAKI ASIAN NOODLES

C | 187
F | 3.5g

SUPER-QUICK, super-fresh, and super-healthy.

Yield:	Prep time:
4 servings	about 2 minutes

Ingredients:

8 tablespoons sugar-free teriyaki sauce (such as Seal Sama)

2 tablespoons chopped, no-added-sugar hot-pickled cherry peppers plus 2 tablespoons pickling liquid (such as Delallo)

16 ounces tofu shirataki spaghetti, rinsed, drained, and roughly cut to 4-inch pieces

5 cups broccoli slaw (such as Dole)

12 ounces roasted, store-bought chicken, skin removed and shredded

Method:

1. *Mix* the teriyaki sauce, pickled peppers, and pickling liquid in a large mixing bowl. *Add* the remaining ingredients and *mix* to evenly coat everything with the sauce.

2. Place the salad evenly onto 4 salad plates.

Tip:

- Add ¼ cup cilantro sprigs to each portion for a fresh boost of flavor with no added calories.

Per serving:

187 calories, 3.5g fat (0.7g sat), 75.75mg cholesterol, 741mg sodium, 11.25g carbohydrates, 4g fiber, 30.2g protein

Nutrient content claims:

Reduced calorie / Reduced fat / Low saturated fat / No added sugar / Good source of fiber / High protein / Trans fat free

Recommended ready-made version:
Weight Watchers Smart Ones Thai Style Chicken and Noodles with Carrots
Calories: 260 / Fat: 4g

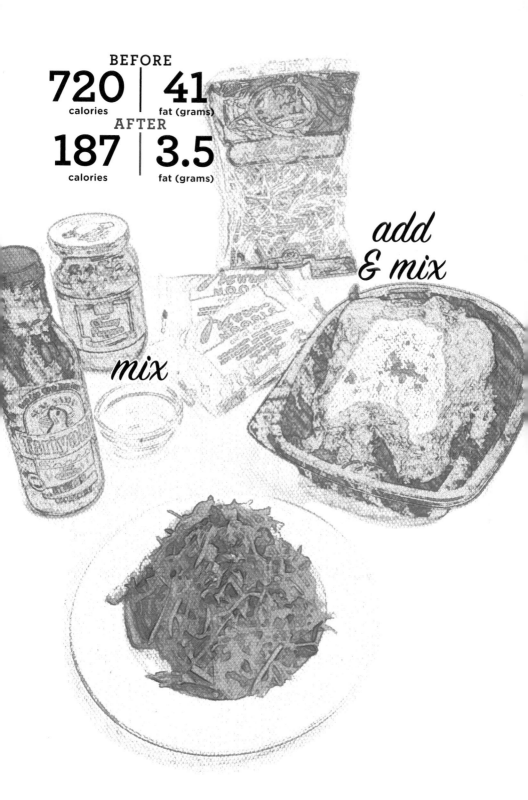

BEFORE

720 calories | **41** fat (grams)

AFTER

187 calories | **3.5** fat (grams)

mix

add & mix

THAI NOODLES WITH TURKEY

C | 199
F | 8g

GREAT AUTHENTIC FLAVOR quicker than takeout. Using the ultimate in low-calorie-density shirataki noodles and a metabolism-boosting spicy red curry paste, this dish is a snap to prepare. The fat content of peanut butter is similar to that of olive oil (good fat!) and it also has a good amount of potassium, which helps regulate the sodium levels in your body. The sauce element of this recipe can make eating healthy raw veggies an addiction!

Yield:	Prep time:	Cooking time:
4 servings	about 5 minutes	about 5 minutes

Ingredients:

¼   cup no-added-sugar-or-salt peanut butter (such as Smucker's Natural)

2   teaspoons no-added-sugar red curry paste (panang paste)

½   cup water

Olive oil cooking spray (such as Pam)

16   ounces shirataki spaghetti, rinsed, drained, and cut roughly into 4-to-5-inch pieces

3¾   cups frozen sliced mixed bell peppers and onions (such as Birds Eye Pepper and Onion Stir-Fry)

6   ounces sliced turkey breast, sliced ¼ inch thick at deli

Salt and crushed red pepper flakes

Method:

1. *Whisk* the peanut butter, red curry paste, and water in a medium-sized mixing bowl until well incorporated and saucelike, about 30 seconds.

2. *Spray* a nonstick skillet with 4 seconds of cooking spray and place over medium-high heat. Add the noodles and *cook* until all the water has evaporated. *Add* the pepper and onion mixture and the turkey and *cook* over medium-high heat until the vegetables are tender and their liquid has mostly evaporated, about 1 minute. *Add* the sauce to the skillet and toss until everything is coated and hot. *Season* to taste with salt and red pepper flakes. Using tongs, evenly divide the contents of the skillet among four plates and serve.

Tips:

- This is a great cold noodle salad dish as well; just chill after making it and keep it in the refrigerator for up to 3 days.
- You can add a fresh burst of cilantro to the dish for next to no calories.

Per serving:

199 calories, 8g fat (1g sat), 35.25mg cholesterol, 109.5mg sodium, 10g carbohydrate, 2.5g fiber, 17.75g protein

Nutrient content claims:

Reduced calorie / Reduced fat / Low saturated fat / Low sodium / No added sugar / High protein / Trans fat free / Gluten free / Good source of fiber

Recommended ready-made version:

Weight Watchers Smart Ones Thai Style Chicken and Rice Noodles

Calories: 260 / Fat: 4g

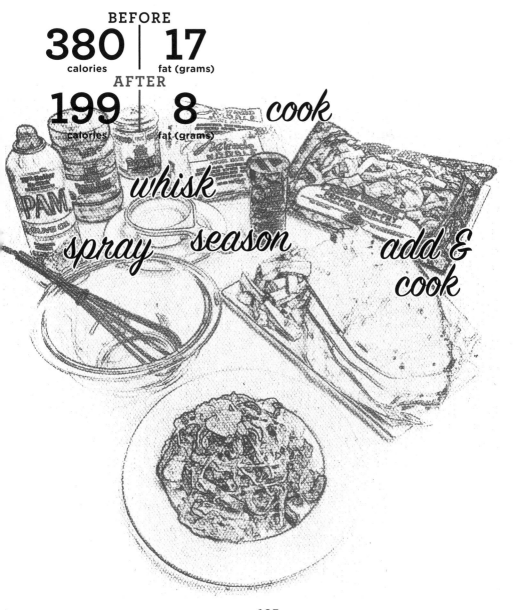

BEFORE

380 | **17**

calories | fat (grams)

AFTER

199 | **8**

calories | fat (grams)

cook

whisk

spray *season* *add & cook*

TURKEY ALFREDO

C | 206
F | 3.5g

THIS IS MY VERSION of the ever-emulated chicken Alfredo. These noodles have a tenth of the calories of normal pasta and are made primarily of dietary fiber, so you can eat them guilt free. The texture of the sauce comes from the magical hydrocolloid called xanthan gum, so this insanely low-calorie pasta dish is entirely gluten free!

Yield:	Prep time:	Cooking time:
4 servings	about 1 minute	about 5 minutes

Ingredients:

2 **cups fat-free milk**
1 **ounce Pecorino Romano cheese, grated**
1/2 **teaspoon xanthan gum (such as Bob's Red Mill)**
   Salt and freshly ground black pepper
16 **ounces tofu shirataki fettuccine noodles, rinsed under cold water, drained, and cut roughly into 4-to-5-inch pieces**
12 **ounces 1/4-inch-thick sliced store-roasted turkey breast**

Method:

1. Combine the milk in a blender and *blend* on low. *Add* three-quarters of the cheese and *blend* until smooth. With the blender still on low, *sprinkle* in the xanthan gum and continue to *blend* until the mixture has thickened to a saucelike texture. *Season* with salt and pepper and set aside.

2. Place a large nonstick skillet over medium-high heat, add the noodles, and *cook* until they're very hot and the water has evaporated from the bottom of the skillet. *Add* the turkey and the sauce to the skillet and *cook* until the mixture is hot and the noodles are coated with the sauce.

3. Adjust the seasoning and, using tongs, evenly divide the pasta among four bowls. Sprinkle the remaining cheese evenly over the four dishes and serve.

Tips:

- Replace all or some of the turkey with your favorite low-calorie-density food, like broccoli, and save 20 calories per each ounce of turkey replaced with the vegetable.
- To boost umami flavor, add 1 1/2 teaspoons yeast flakes (such as Red Star) for an additional 6 calories per portion.

Per serving:

206 calories, 3.5g fat (1.2g sat), 80.25mg cholesterol, 245.5mg sodium, 62.8g carbohydrate, 2.3g fiber, 32.4g protein

Nutrient content claims:

Reduced calorie / Reduced fat / No sugar added / High protein / Trans fat free / Gluten free

BEFORE

1,220 | **75**
calories | fat (grams)

AFTER

206 | **3.5**
calories | fat (grams)

sprinkle

*add &
blend*

*add &
cook*

season

SALISBURY STEAK WITH MUSHROOM GRAVY

C | 178
F | 6g

I LOVE THIS RECIPE because with the great lean beef out there, when you decide to eat beef you can really take control of the fat content. Using the low-calorie-density mushrooms really carries the beef's flavor and texture while filling you up, so you can use less of the calorie-rich beef. Make sure the patties aren't thick or they'll take too long to cook.

Yield:	Prep time:	Cooking time:
4 servings	about 1 minute	about 5 minutes

Ingredients:

Olive oil cooking spray (such as Pam)

12 ounces 96% lean ground beef (such as Laura's Lean)

Salt and freshly ground black pepper

½ cup unsalted beef stock (such as Kitchen Basics)

½ cup 98% fat-free cream of mushroom soup (such as Campbell's)

2 cups (8 ounces) tofu shirataki macaroni (or substitute another shirataki noodle cut), rinsed and dried

3 ounces 75% reduced-fat cheddar cheese (such as Cabot), grated

Method:

1. *Spray* a large nonstick skillet with 4 seconds of cooking spray and place over medium-high heat. *Form* the beef into 4 patties about ½ inch thick, *season* with salt and pepper, and *brown* on one side of the patties, about 1 minute. Flip the patties and brown the other side, about another minute. *Add* the stock and soup, bring to a *simmer*, and *cook* until done to your liking, about 2 minutes for medium rare.

2. Place the noodles in a small saucepot with 2 tablespoons of water, bring to a *boil* over medium heat, and *add* the cheese. *Stir* over medium heat until a sauce forms, season with salt and pepper, and divide among four plates. Place a steak on each plate and spoon the remaining sauce over the top.

Tip:

- You can cook the noodles and cheese ahead of time and just reheat in the microwave.

Per serving:

178 calories, 6g fat (2.75g sat), 52.5mg cholesterol, 433.25mg sodium, 3.9g carbohydrate, 1.25g fiber, 26g protein

Nutrient content claims:

Reduced calorie / Reduced fat / No added sugar / High protein / Trans fat free

BEFORE

440 calories | **32** fat (grams)

AFTER

178 calories | **6** fat (grams)

spray

*add &
simmer*

*form,
season,
& brown*

*boil &
stir*

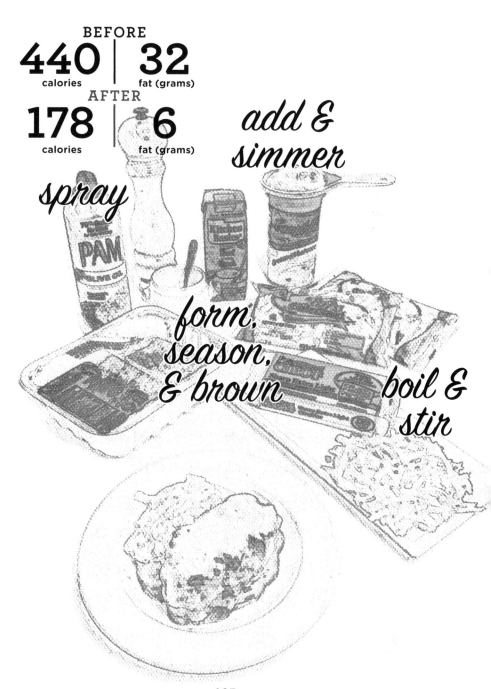

SALISBURY STEAK WITH MUSHROOM GRAVY

LEMON GARLIC SHRIMP PASTA

C | 105
F | 1g

SHRIMP seem to have a bad rep with those who fear high cholesterol. Shrimp are relatively high in cholesterol; however, we now know that dietary cholesterol may not impact blood cholesterol the way we once thought it did. Shrimp are also low in saturated fat, which makes them a healthier protein choice than most meats. Shrimp are very low in calories, and since they're so commonly available already boiled in the fish department at the supermarket, or in the freezer section, they're extremely good for quick preparations. Zucchini offers such a nice texture along with its low calorie density, you'll wonder where else to fit it into your cooking. By pairing it with a noodle like the shirataki noodle, which requires no boiling, this high-flavored dish can be made so quickly, with such great results, that it will truly blow your mind.

Yield:	Prep time:	Cooking time:
4 servings	about 2 minutes	about 5 minutes

Ingredients:

Olive oil cooking spray (such as Pam)

2   tablespoons plus 2 teaspoons chopped garlic

Crushed red pepper flakes

2   cups organic zucchini, washed and cut into ½-inch half-moons

16   ounces shirataki spaghetti, rinsed under cold water, drained, and roughly cut into 4-to-5-inch pieces

12   ounces peeled and cooked domestic white shrimp

¼   cup fresh lemon juice

Salt

Method:

1. *Spray* a large nonstick skillet with 4 seconds of olive oil spray and place over medium-high heat. *Add* the garlic and *cook*, stirring, until it turns a deep golden brown color. *Add* a pinch of red pepper flakes and the zucchini and *cook* until the zucchini is warmed through and softened, about 2 minutes. *Add* the noodles and shrimp and let the excess water *evaporate* while stirring.

2. Once the water has evaporated, *add* the lemon juice and turn off the heat. *Season with salt.* Evenly divide the pasta among four plates and serve.

Tip:

- Use domestic white or pink shrimp when possible; many of the farmed southeast Asian varieties taste a little muddy.

Per serving:

105 calories, 1g fat (0g sat), 165.75mg cholesterol, 197mg sodium, 5g carbohydrate, 2g fiber, 19g protein

Nutrient content claims:

Reduced calorie / Low fat / Saturated fat free / No added sugar / High protein / Trans fat free / Gluten free

Recommended ready-made version:

Lean Cuisine Culinary Collection Lemon Garlic Shrimp

Calories: 280 / Fat: 6g

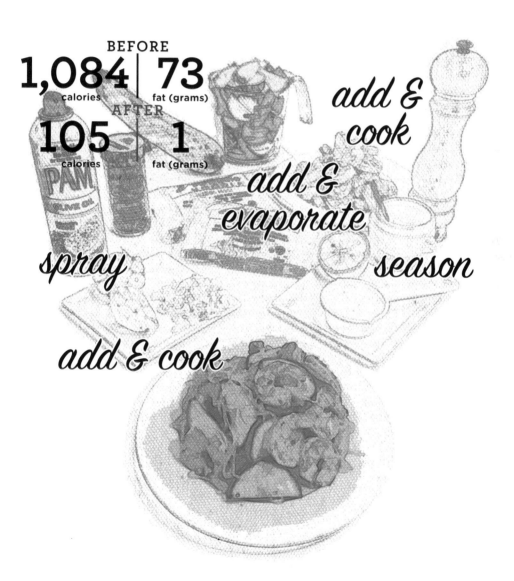

BEFORE

1,084 | **73**
calories | fat (grams)

AFTER

105 | **1**
calories | fat (grams)

add & cook

add & evaporate

spray

season

add & cook

BEEF AND BROCCOLI STIR-FRY

C | 193
F | 4g

THIS IS A GOOD example of a perfectly healthy dish that has gone awry. What could be a nice healthy entree has been clobbered by sugar, starch, and sickened beef. Here I have taken the classic beef with broccoli, A DISH I LOVE, and made a few changes that cut unneeded fat calories by simply inverting the ratios of beef and broccoli. You still have all the rich beef flavor to coat the broccoli, which satisfies the craving for this stir-fry, but without any more beef than is really necessary. Use grass-fed beef here, as the flavor will stand out more so you can use less.

Yield:	Prep time:	Processing time:
4 servings	about 2 minutes	about 5 minutes

Ingredients:

Olive oil cooking spray (such as Pam)

12 ounces grass-fed beef tenderloin, sliced into ¼-inch strips

Salt and freshly ground black pepper

6 cups frozen broccoli florets, defrosted

2 cups shirataki rice, rinsed and drained (such as Miracle Noodle—substitute a different shirataki product and chop it up if the rice cut is unavailable)

1 cup cold water

2 tablespoons plus 2 teaspoons instant brown gravy (such as Knorr) mixed with 1 cup cold water

6 tablespoons reduced-sodium sugar-free teriyaki sauce (such as Seal Sama)

Method:

1. *Spray* a large nonstick skillet with 2 seconds of cooking spray and place over high heat. *Season* the beef with salt and pepper. Place half the meat in the skillet and *brown* one side evenly, about 1 minute. *Remove* the browned beef and set aside. Spray the skillet with 2 seconds of cooking spray and repeat with the remaining beef.

2. Spray the skillet with 2 seconds of cooking spray, then *add* the broccoli and rice and *cook* until all the water has evaporated, about 1 minute. *Add* the water-gravy mixture and teriyaki sauce to the pan and *simmer* until thickened to a saucelike texture, about 10 seconds.

3. *Season* with salt and pepper, then divide the stir-fry among four bowls and serve.

Tip:
• Add some crushed red pepper flakes if you want to spice things up a bit.

Per serving:
193 calories, 4g fat (1.5g sat), 60mg cholesterol, 763mg sodium, 11g carbohydrate, 3g fiber, 26g protein

BEFORE

720 | **24**
calories | fat (grams)

AFTER

193 | **4**
calories | fat (grams)

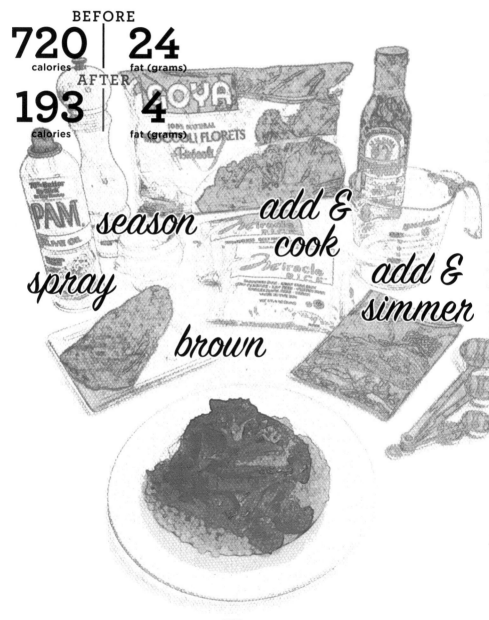

spray

season

brown

add &
cook

add &
simmer

BEEF AND BROCCOLI STIR-FRY

ROASTED TURKEY WITH GREEN BEANS AND GRAVY

C | 138
F | 1g

I LOVE TURKEY and gravy—the flavors remind me of Thanksgiving gluttony and the belly-rubbing satiated feeling that comes with it. Here is a super-fast recipe that swaps out mashed potatoes for high-fiber gravy-grabbing green beans, adds dried cranberries for excitement, and uses oven-roasted turkey that heats extremely well in this instant gravy.

Yield:	Prep time:	Cooking time:
4 servings	about 1 minute	about 5 minutes

Ingredients:

1   tablespoon salt
4   cups green beans, stems trimmed
1   cup water
2   tablespoons plus 2 teaspoons poultry gravy mix (such as Knorr Roasted Chicken)
8   ounces store-roasted turkey breast, skin removed, sliced ¼ inch thick at deli
    Salt and freshly ground black pepper
2   tablespoons dried cranberries

Method:

1. Bring 2 quarts of water to a boil in a wide saucepot. Add the tablespoon of salt, drop the beans in, and *cook* until tender but still retaining some vitality, about 3 minutes. *Strain* the beans, drain the water out of the pot, and keep the beans *warm* in the pot on the stove with no heat.

2. Pour the 1 cup water into a large high-sided skillet and *whisk* in the gravy mix until fully incorporated. Turn to medium-high heat and bring the gravy to a *simmer*, whisking, until it becomes thick. *Add* the turkey, stir to *coat* it with the gravy, and turn off the heat.

3. *Season* the beans with salt and pepper and divide them among four plates. Evenly divide the turkey among the plates next to the beans and spoon the remaining sauce over the turkey. *Sprinkle* the cranberries over each dish and serve.

Per serving:
138 calories, 1g fat (0g sat), 47mg cholesterol, 237mg sodium, 13g carbohydrate, 3.6g fiber, 19.5g protein

Nutrient content claims:
Reduced calorie / Low fat / Saturated fat free / Good source of fiber / High protein

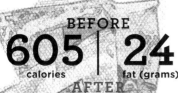

BEFORE

605 | 24

calories | fat (grams)

AFTER

138 | 1

calories | fat (grams)

add & coat with sauce

whisk & simmer

cook, strain, & keep warm

season

sprinkle

SWEET SESAME TURKEY WITH BOK CHOY

C | 147
F | 2g

BY USING TURKEY instead of the ubiquitous chicken, I immediately save calories in this delicious stir-fry. I also employ the cruciferous and high-water-content Chinese cabbage called bok choy, which is a high-volume, low-calorie food—meaning it fills you up without weighing you down. The small, sweet, tender leaves and stalks can be enjoyed with just a little bit of cooking, which makes them very handy when you're watching your minutes as well as your calories.

Yield:	Prep time:	Cooking time:
4 servings	about 2 minutes	about 3 minutes

Ingredients:

Olive oil cooking spray (such as Pam)

12 ounces cooked turkey breast, cut into 1/2-inch dice

2 cups shirataki rice, rinsed and drained (such as Miracle Noodle—substitute a different shirataki product and chop it up if the rice cut is unavailable)

Salt and crushed red pepper flakes

5 cups bok choy, roughly chopped into bite-sized pieces

6 tablespoons reduced-sodium sugar-free teriyaki sauce (such as Seal Sama)

1 tablespoon toasted sesame seeds

Method:

1. *Spray* a large nonstick skillet with 2 seconds of olive oil spray and place over high heat. Add the turkey and *cook* until *brown* on all sides (about 1 minute); *add* the rice and salt and pepper flakes to taste and *cook* until hot, about 1 minute. Transfer the mixture to a bowl and set aside.

2. Spray the skillet with 2 seconds of olive oil spray, put the bok choy in the skillet, and *cook* until the vegetables are just wilted and barely warmed through, about 1 minute. Put the turkey and rice mixture back in the skillet, *add* the teriyaki sauce, and *toss* together until everything has sauce adhering to it. Spoon evenly into four bowls and sprinkle each bowl with sesame seeds.

Per serving:

147 calories, 2g fat (0g sat), 70.5mg cholesterol, 551.5mg sodium, 4g carbohydrate, 1g fiber, 29g protein

Nutrient content claims:

Reduced calorie / Low fat / Saturated fat free / No added sugar / High protein / Trans fat free

Recommended ready-made version:
Lean Cuisine Spa Collection Sesame Stir-Fry with Chicken
Calories: 290 / Fat: 7g

BEFORE
640 | **6**
calories | fat (grams)

AFTER
147 | **2**
calories | fat (grams)

cook

*add &
cook*

sprinkle

spray

*cook &
brown*

VEGETABLE EGG ROLLS WITH CHIA-CHILI SAUCE

C | 192
F | 1.5g

WHO DOESN'T LOVE an egg roll? I bet you didn't know you could make a fat-free, low-calorie version of this cravable classic in the same amount of time it takes for the delivery to reach your door! The slaw made of the cruciferous vegetables cabbage and broccoli offers a great stomach filler with very few caloric ramifications, and these veggies have been shown to stop the growth of some cancer cells—now, that's a deal! I use the nutrient-rich chia seed to thicken this dipping sauce, avoiding high-sugar syrupy thickeners and high-carb processed starch thickeners.

Yield:	Prep time:	Cooking time:
4 servings	about 1 minute	about 5 minutes

Ingredients:

1	tablespoon plus 1 teaspoon chia seeds
¼	cup water
	Olive oil cooking spray (such as Pam)
8	cups broccoli and vegetable slaw (such as Dole)
¼	cup plus 1 tablespoon reduced-sodium sugar-free teriyaki sauce (such as Seal Sama)
	Salt and freshly ground black pepper
8	egg roll wrappers (in the refrigerated section of the supermarket, usually by the tofu)
2	tablespoons chili garlic paste (such as Lan Chi)

Method:

1. Preheat the oven to 450°F. In a small mixing bowl, *mix* the chia seeds with the water and set aside. Spray a very large nonstick skillet with cooking spray and place it over high heat. Once the skillet is hot, add the slaw and *cook* until the vegetables have softened, about 1 minute. *Add* 2 tablespoons of the teriyaki sauce to the skillet and cook until it sticks to the slaw, then remove the mixture to a mixing bowl and *season* with salt and pepper.

2. Place aluminum foil shiny side up on a cookie sheet, then place a wire rack over the sheet. Place the wrappers on a clean surface, divide the vegetables among them, and *wrap* as shown on the package. Set on the rack and spray with 2 seconds of cooking spray. Place in the oven and *cook* until lightly browned and crispy, about 3 minutes.

3. *Mix* the remaining teriyaki sauce into the chia seed mixture with the chili paste and spoon evenly into four dipping dishes. Place two egg rolls each on four plates and serve with the sauce.

Tip:

- If you have trouble closing the ends of your eggrolls, don't sweat it—they're not going in the fryer anyway, so just be careful not to let the mixture spill out of the ends when you're handling them.

Per serving:

192 calories, 1.5g fat (0g sat), 6.75 mg cholesterol, 837.25mg sodium, 30.5g carbohydrate, 6.5g fiber, 11g protein

Nutrient content claims:

Reduced calorie / Low fat / Saturated fat free / Low cholesterol / High fiber / High protein / Trans fat free

> *Recommended ready-made version:*
> Lean Cuisine Simple Favorites Vegetable Eggrolls
> Calories: 320 / Fat: 4g

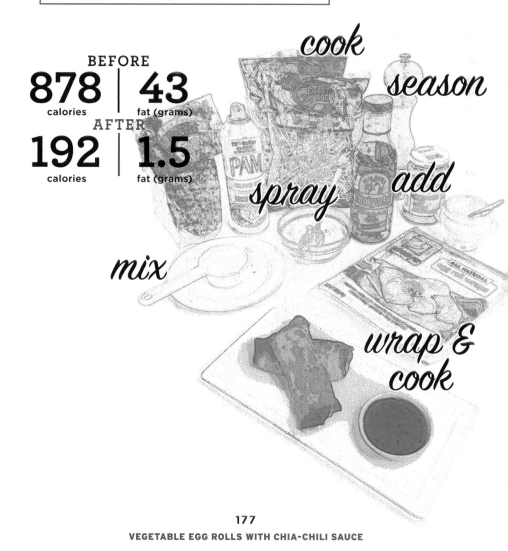

BEFORE

878 | **43**
calories | fat (grams)

AFTER

192 | **1.5**
calories | fat (grams)

cook

season

spray

add

mix

wrap & cook

VEGETABLE EGG ROLLS WITH CHIA-CHILI SAUCE

PORK CUTLET ALLA PIZZAIOLA

C | 193
F | 3g

SIMPLY TRANSLATED "meat and tomato sauce," this dish originated in Naples as a way to make less expensive cuts of meat tender by cooking for a long time in tomato sauce. Our lives are a bit busier now than back then, but we still like less expensive, so in my version we get flavorful, tender, less expensive, and quick by using fast cooking and delicious pork tenderloin. This dish will suit the critics in the family, and by using beans, I can offer a gluten-free (and classic) alternative to pasta with tomato sauce as well as no dairy. Nice!

Yield:	Prep time:	Processing time:
4 servings	about 1 minute	about 5 minutes

Ingredients:

Olive oil cooking spray (such as Pam)

4 pork cutlets, 2½ ounces each

Salt and freshly ground black pepper

5 cloves garlic, sliced very thin

14-ounce bag frozen pepper and onion mix (such as Birds Eye Pepper and Onion Stir-Fry)

2 cups no-added-salt-or-sugar whole peeled plum tomatoes

1 cup drained reduced-sodium white cannellini beans (such as Eden)

Method:

1. *Spray* a large nonstick skillet with 2 seconds of cooking spray and place over high heat. *Season* each side of the cutlets with salt and pepper. Place the cutlets in the skillet and *brown* each side evenly, about 1 minute per side. *Remove* the browned cutlets and set aside.

2. Add the garlic to the skillet and *cook* until deep golden brown, about 1 minute. *Add* the pepper and onion mixture, tomatoes, and beans and bring to a *simmer*. Add the pork cutlets and cook until cooked through, 2 to 4 minutes. Place the entire contents of the skillet on a large serving dish and serve family style.

Tips:

• Remove the pork from the refrigerator 30 minutes in advance for quick and even cooking.

• Add some crushed red pepper flakes if you want to spice things up a bit.

Per serving:

193 calories, 3g fat (.94g sat), 34.25mg cholesterol, 318.75mg sodium, 20.25g carbohydrate, 4.5g fiber, 20.5g protein

BEFORE

878
calories

43
fat (grams)

AFTER

193
calories

3
fat (grams)

season

add & simmer

brown & remove

spray

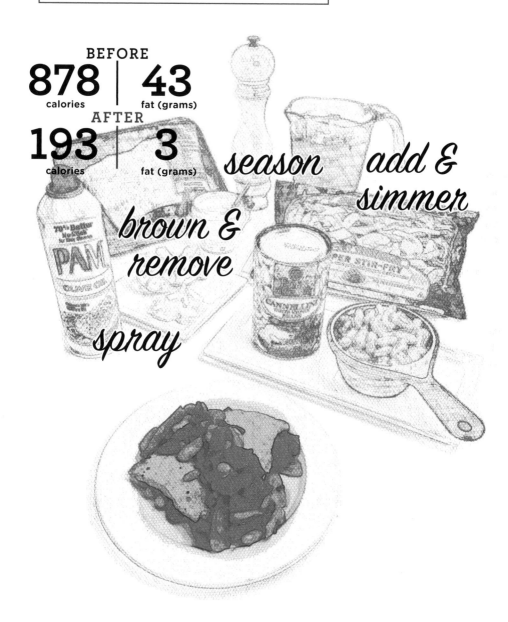

RD'S BIG BURGER WITH ALL THE FIXIN'S

C | 215
F | 4.5g

THIS TOOK QUITE a while in my test kitchen, but it was time well spent. It's a great burger experience for a fraction of the usual fat and calories. Often, calorie-dense foods are just vehicles for other flavors that people associate with a particular dish. By using a controlled amount of 96 percent lean ground beef and adding volume with puffed brown rice and water, I have created a filling patty that is a vehicle for the classic flavors of a "special sauce," albeit fat free and reduced sugar of course. Add some no-sugar-added pickles and fat-free American cheese and you will have a 100 percent legitimate burger experience for 65 percent fewer calories and almost 90 percent less fat.

Yield:	Prep time:	Cooking time:
4 servings	about 3 minutes	about 3 minutes

Ingredients:

1	cup puffed rice
1/4	cup cold water
12	ounces 96% lean ground beef (such as Laura's Lean)
	Salt and freshly ground black pepper
	Olive oil cooking spray (such as Pam)
1 1/2	tablespoons reduced-sugar ketchup (such as Heinz)
4 1/2	tablespoons fat-free mayonnaise (such as Kraft)
4	low-calorie hamburger buns (such as Sara Lee Delightful Wheat)

Method:

1. In a food processor, *process* the puffed rice until it's broken up, about 10 seconds. Add the water and *mix* until all the water is absorbed into the rice, about 10 seconds. Add the ground beef and *process* until evenly incorporated. Working on squares of wax paper, *form* the mixture into 4 patties about 5 inches in diameter and season the tops with salt and pepper.

2. *Spray* a large nonstick skillet with 2 seconds of cooking spray and place over high heat. Turn the patties into the skillet, peel the paper off the top of each patty, and season with salt and pepper. *Brown* each side until cooked through, about 1 1/2 minutes per side.

3. Meanwhile, *mix* the ketchup and mayonnaise in a small bowl and set aside. Place each patty on a bun, *top* each patty evenly with the sauce, choose your toppings (see below), and serve.

Tips:

• If you like your buns toasted, place the buns cut side down in the skillet before you cook the patties.

- Keep the patties cold before cooking; they'll be easier to handle.
- Use unsalted chicken stock instead of the water for a little flavor boost.
- Optional garnish: Make a personalized burger with these health-friendly options:
  - Up to 8 slices dill hamburger pickles (such as Heinz) for 0 calories
  - Iceberg lettuce leaves for only 1 calorie per whole leaf
  - Fresh tomato slices for 3 calories per slice
  - 1 slice of fat-free cheese for 25 calories

Per serving:
215 calories, 4.5g fat (1.5g), 47mg cholesterol, 422mg sodium, 20g carbohydrate, 6g fiber, 22g protein

Nutrient content claims:
Reduced calorie / Reduced fat / No added sugar / High fiber / High protein / Trans fat free

Recommended ready-made version:
Lean Pockets Cheese Burger
Calories: 290 / Fat: 9g

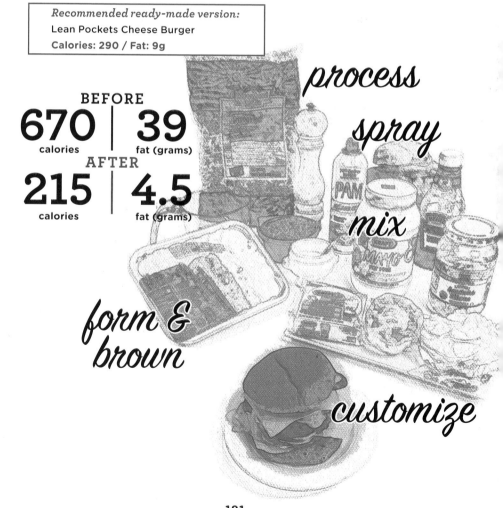

BEFORE
670 | 39
calories | fat (grams)

AFTER
215 | 4.5
calories | fat (grams)

process

spray

mix

form & brown

customize

BACON-WRAPPED CHICKEN WITH SWEET RUTABAGA MASH

C | 232
F | 4g

A HIGH-PROTEIN dinner with a delicious alternative to mashed potatoes. Low-calorie-density rutabaga is the sweet star in this recipe.

Yield:	Prep time:	Cooking time:
4 servings	about 2 minutes	about 5 minutes

Ingredients:

4   boneless, skinless chicken cutlets (4 ounces each)
     Salt and freshly ground black pepper
8   slices lean turkey bacon (such as Butterball Everyday Thin & Crispy)
1   tablespoon raw agave nectar
3   packets monk fruit extract (such as Monk Fruit In The Raw)
4   cups peeled and roughly grated rutabaga

Method:

1. Place a rack 10 inches under the broiler and preheat. *Season* each side of the chicken cutlets with salt and pepper. *Wrap* each cutlet with two strips of bacon lengthwise, folding any excess bacon under the cutlet. Place the wrapped cutlets bacon side up on a sheet tray fitted with a wire rack and place under the broiler to *brown* the bacon and *cook* the chicken through, about 5 minutes.

2. Meanwhile, *mix* the agave nectar and monk fruit extract in a small bowl and stir to combine. Place the rutabaga in a microwave-safe bowl with the agave and monk fruit extract mixture, *cover* with wax or parchment paper, and *cook* on high until very tender, about 5 minutes. Remove the paper and season with salt.

3. Evenly divide the rutabaga among four plates, place a chicken breast next to each dollop of rutabaga, and serve.

Tip:

- Try adding a pinch of curry powder to the rutabaga while it cooks; it's very good with the sweetness of the vegetable, and the turmeric in the curry is extremely good for you.

Per serving:
232 calories, 4g fat (.925g sat), 80.5mg cholesterol, 288.5mg sodium, 18g carbohydrate, 4.5g fiber, 31g protein

Nutrient content claims:
Reduced calorie / Reduced fat / Low saturated fat / Good source of fiber / High protein / Gluten free / Trans fat free

BEFORE

638 calories | **51** fat (grams)

AFTER

232 calories | **4** fat (grams)

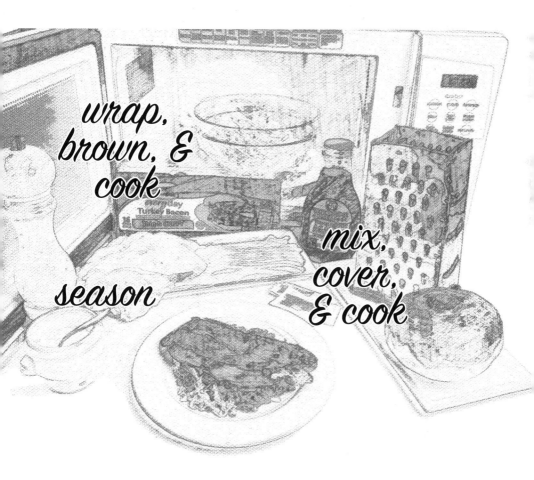

wrap, brown, & cook

mix, cover, & cook

season

BACON-WRAPPED CHICKEN WITH SWEET RUTABAGA MASH

BBQ CHICKEN CUTLETS

C | 129
F | 1g

I LIKE THIS dish because it can be assembled in minutes. The chicken is precut, and the sauce is just mixed in a bowl and brushed right on. With calories this low, you can afford to eat these as a snack!

Yield:	Prep time:	Cooking time:
4 servings	about 2 minutes	about 5 minutes

Ingredients:

Olive oil cooking spray (such as Pam)

16 ounces chicken breast cutlets

Salt and freshly ground black pepper

3 tablespoons reduced-sugar ketchup (such as Heinz)

1 tablespoon red wine vinegar

1 teaspoon liquid smoke

1/2 teaspoon monk fruit extract (such as Monk Fruit In The Raw)

Method:

1. Heat a grill or grill pan over high heat. Spray a kitchen towel with the cooking spray and *rub* over the clean grates of the grill. *Season* both sides of the chicken cutlets with salt and pepper. Once the grill is hot, *grill* the cutlets on one side for 1 minute. Flip the cutlets.

2. Meanwhile, in a small bowl *whisk* together the ketchup, vinegar, liquid smoke, and monk fruit extract until smooth. Season to taste with salt and pepper.

3. *Brush* the tops of the cutlets with some of the sauce. Continue to grill for 1 minute. Flip the cutlets once more and brush the tops with the remaining sauce. Flip and move the cutlets until the sauce is caramelized on both sides and the chicken is no longer pink. Transfer the chicken to a platter and serve.

Per serving:

129 calories, 1g fat (0g sat), 65.75mg cholesterol, 204mg sodium, 0.75g carbohydrate, 0g fiber, 26g protein

Nutrient content claims:

Reduced calorie / Low fat / Saturated fat free / Trans fat free / High protein / Gluten free / No added sugar

> *Recommended ready-made version:*
> Lean Cuisine Culinary Collection Chile Lime Chicken
> **Calories: 240 / Fat: 2g**

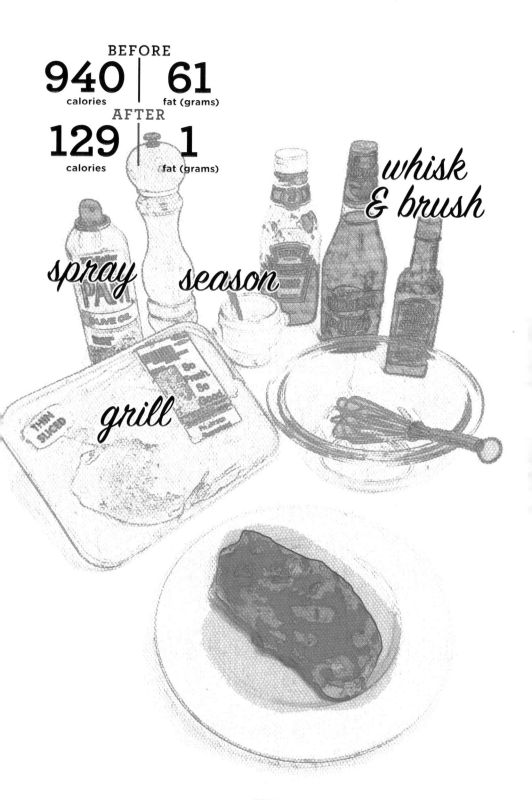

BEFORE

940 | **61**

calories | fat (grams)

AFTER

129 | **1**

calories | fat (grams)

spray

season

whisk & brush

grill

185

BBQ CHICKEN CUTLETS

CHICKEN CHEESESTEAK WITH JALAPEÑOS

C | 180
F | 5.5g

GOTTA FEEL LIKE you're really eating sometimes, ya know? Like getting a little messy and really eating. I designed this dish to deliver a true cheesesteak experience that is very low in calories and is based on the metabolism-boosting capsicum of chili peppers!

Yield:	Prep time:	Cooking time:
4 servings	about 1 minute	about 5 minutes

Ingredients:

Olive oil cooking spray (such as Pam)

2 low-calorie whole-wheat hot dog buns (such as Sara Lee Delightful Wheat), split into 4 long pieces

12 ounces shaved chicken (such as Old Neighborhood)

Salt and freshly ground black pepper

¼ cup chopped pickled jalapeños

2 cups frozen pepper and onion mix (such as Birds Eye Pepper and Onion Stir-Fry)

2 ounces 75% reduced-fat cheddar cheese (such as Cabot)

Method:

1. *Spray* a large nonstick skillet with 2 seconds of cooking spray and place over high heat. Put the buns in the skillet cut side down and *toast* until golden brown, about 1 minute. Remove them, place half a bun on each of four plates, and return the skillet to the stove.

2. *Season* the chicken with salt and pepper, place in the hot skillet, and *cook* through, stirring, about 1 minute. *Add* the jalapeños and the pepper and onion mixture and *cook* until the water has evaporated. *Season* with salt and pepper.

3. *Sprinkle* in the cheese and fold the mixture together until the cheese begins to *melt* and form a sauce with the liquid from the peppers, about 30 seconds. Place an equal amount on the cut side of each roll and serve.

Per serving:

180 calories, 5.5g fat (2.25g sat), 57.5mg cholesterol, 345.34mg sodium, 10.505g carbohydrate, 2.325g fiber, 22.67g protein

Nutrient content claims:

Reduced calorie / Reduced fat / High protein / No added sugar / Trans fat free

Recommended ready-made version:
Lean Cuisine Culinary Collection Philly Style Steak & Cheese Panini
Calories: 320 / Fat: 9g

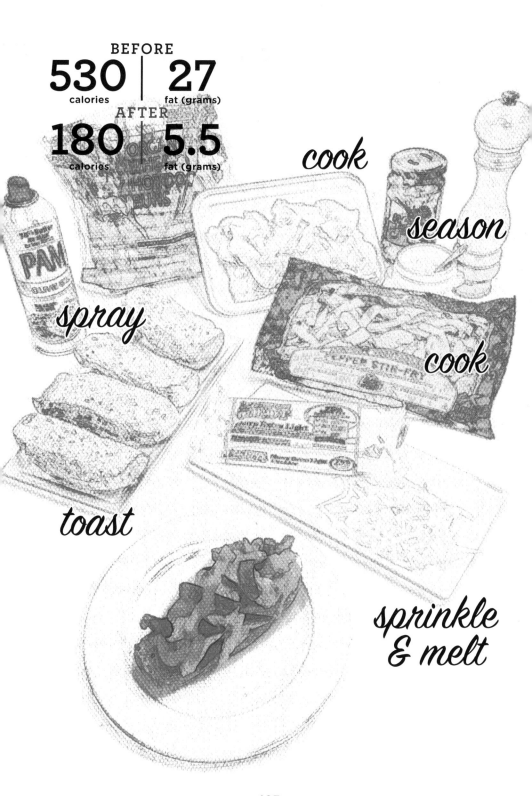

BEFORE

530 calories | **27** fat (grams)

AFTER

180 calories | **5.5** fat (grams)

cook

season

spray

cook

toast

sprinkle & melt

CHICKEN CHEESESTEAK WITH JALAPEÑOS

CHICKEN ENCHILADAS

C 225
F 6.5g

I LIKE THIS DISH because it serves as a good template for many quick-dish ideas. I did all the heavy lifting here (no, this is not an excuse for you to skip your workout!) so I could provide all of us with different tastes—a way to enjoy a dish that is usually a deceptively high-calorie one. Keep your metabolism moving with a spicy pico de gallo here, and use fat-free yogurt mixed with lime juice as a fat-free sour cream replacement in your other dishes that may call for whole sour cream.

Yield:	Prep time:	Cooking time:
4 servings	about 1 minute	about 5 minutes

Ingredients:

8   ounces roasted boneless, skinless chicken, shredded (take the skin off a preroasted bird from your supermarket)

1   cup store-bought pico de gallo, at room temperature (such as Ready Pac—as spicy as you can take it!)

    Salt and freshly ground black pepper

8   low-carb tortillas (such as La Tortilla Factory)

1   ounce 75% reduced-fat cheddar cheese (such as Cabot)

½   cup fat-free Greek yogurt (such as Fage Total 0%)

4   lime wedges for serving

Method:

1. *Combine* the chicken and the pico de gallo in a small bowl, mix, and *season* with salt and pepper. Lay out the tortillas on a clean surface and spoon the chicken mixture evenly into the center of each tortilla. *Roll* each tortilla up and place in a microwave-safe 13x9x2-inch baking dish. Spoon any remaining pico de gallo over the top of the enchiladas and *sprinkle* evenly with the cheese. *Cook* on high until the enchiladas are warmed through and the cheese is melted, 3 to 4 minutes.

2. Remove the baking dish from the microwave. Using a spatula, place two enchiladas each on four plates, *top* with equal amounts of the yogurt, and *serve* with fresh lime wedges.

Tips:

- You can top each dish with ¼ cup fresh cilantro for only an additional 1 calorie!
- Replace the chicken in this recipe with steamed shrimp and save 19 calories per portion and over half a gram of fat.
- You can use a microwave instead of the oven with similar results: Cook the enchiladas in a microwave-safe dish for 2 minutes on high.

Per serving:
225 calories, 6g fat (.95g sat), 53mg cholesterol, 704mg sodium, 25g carbohydrate, 14g fiber, 31.5g protein

Nutrient content claims:
Reduced calorie / Reduced fat / Low saturated fat / No added sugar / High fiber / High protein / Trans fat free

Recommended ready-made version:
Weight Watchers Smart Ones Chicken Enchiladas Suiza
Calories: 290 / Fat: 5g

BEFORE

530 calories | **27** fat (grams)

AFTER

225 calories | **6.5** fat (grams)

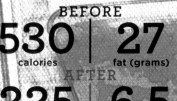

season

roll

combine

sprinkle

top

CRAB TACO WITH PICO DE GALLO AND CILANTRO

C | 144
F | 2g

I LOVE this super-quick recipe because it is not only filling but also can be made without ever picking up a pan or a knife! I bet if you order food for delivery at the same time you start preparing this recipe, you will be done eating my dish by the time the calorically crazy delivery arrives.

Yield:	Prep time:	Cooking time:
4 servings	about 2 minutes	about 3 minutes

Ingredients:

1   cup spicy store-bought salsa or pico de gallo (such as Ready Pac)
8   ounces canned jumbo lump crabmeat
    Olive oil cooking spray (such as Pam)
8   white corn tortillas (such as Mission)
2   cups mixed cabbage slaw (such as Dole)
1   cup fresh cilantro leaves
4   lime wedges for serving

Method:

1. *Mix* the salsa or pico de gallo and crabmeat in a large bowl.

2. *Spray* a nonstick skillet with 1 second of cooking spray and place the skillet over high heat. *Toast* the tortillas over high heat two at a time, about 15 seconds per side, and set aside.

3. Place two tortillas each on four plates and *place* an equal amount of cabbage slaw on top, followed by the crabmeat mixture and the cilantro leaves. *Serve* with the lime wedges.

Per serving:
144 calories, 2g fat (0g sat), 25mg cholesterol, 450mg sodium, 25g carbohydrate, 4g fiber, 9.5g protein

Nutrient content claims:
Reduced calorie / Low fat / Saturated fat free / No added sugar / Good source of fiber / Trans fat free / Gluten free

> *Recommended ready-made version:*
> El Monterey Chicken Taquitos (2 pieces)
> Calories: 170 / Fat: 8g

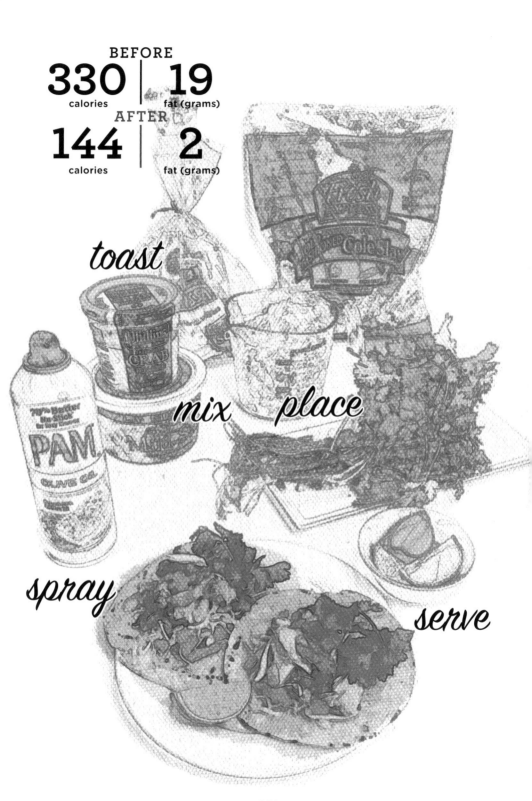

BEFORE

330 | 19
calories | fat (grams)

AFTER

144 | 2
calories | fat (grams)

toast

mix   place

spray

serve

191

CRAB TACO WITH PICO DE GALLO AND CILANTRO

GARLICKY SHRIMP AND SPINACH IN A FOIL POUCH

C | 156
F | 1g

I REALLY LIKE this technique for making super-flavorful dishes in a hurry. Besides the speed, when you cook the ingredients in a sealed vessel, the steam impregnates the dish with the different flavors of every ingredient. It also eliminates the need for fat, not to mention the need to scrub a pan out! This is a protein BOMB—between the great garbanzos, the shrimp, and the spinach, this is packed with goodness.

Yield:	Prep time:	Cooking time:
4 servings	about 2 minutes	about 4 minutes

Ingredients:

- 12 ounces boiled shrimp, shells off
- ½ cup reduced-sodium garbanzo beans, plus ¼ cup of liquid
- 10 ounce box of frozen chopped spinach, thawed
- 2 cups broccoli slaw (such as Dole)
- 3 tablespoons garlic chips (such as Frontier; look in the grocery store spice rack)
-   Salt and crushed red pepper flakes
- 4 lemon wedges for serving

Method:

1. *Lay* four 14-inch pieces of aluminum foil on a work surface.

2. In a bowl, *mix* the first five ingredients together and season with salt and red pepper flakes. Evenly divide the mixture in the center of each piece of foil and *spread* it out so it's not one big pile. *Fold* one corner to the opposite corner, making a triangle, then fold 1 inch of the bottom edge of the foil over the top, seal tightly around all the edges to form four pouches.

3. Heat a 14-inch skillet over high heat. Place two pouches in the skillet and *cook* until they've puffed up, about 1 minute, then remove and place each pouch on a plate. Repeat with the remaining pouches, cut each open, and *serve* with lemon wedges.

Tips:

- Be careful as you cut the pouches open, as the steam is HOT!
- Look in the freezer section for now widely available frozen herbs and add a cube of frozen chopped basil to get an extra flavor boost for 1 additional calorie per serving.

Per serving:
156 calories, 1g fat (0g sat), 166mg cholesterol, 317.5mg sodium, 11g carbohydrate, 3g fiber, 22.25g protein

Recommended ready-made version:

Weight Watchers Smart Ones Shrimp Marinara

Calories: 180 / Fat: 2.5g

BEFORE

460 | **18**

calories | fat (grams)

AFTER

156 | **1**

calories | fat (grams)

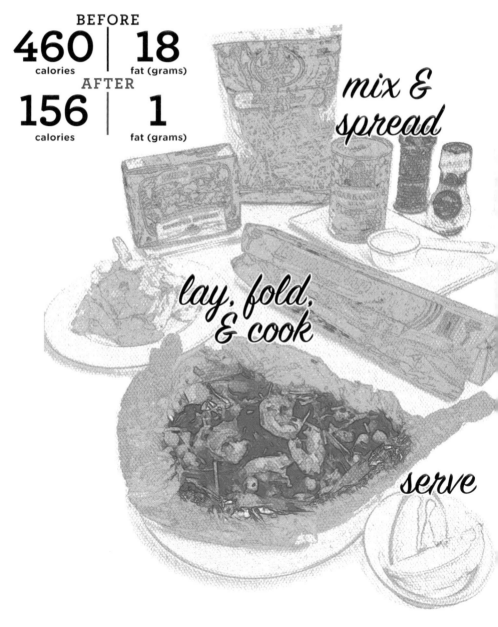

mix & spread

lay, fold, & cook

serve

GARLICKY SHRIMP AND SPINACH IN A FOIL POUCH

ROASTED SCROD WITH VEGETABLE CURRY

C | 199
F | 1.5g

SCROD IS A SMALL haddock, which is very closely related to the overfished Atlantic cod. Choose your fish responsibly by downloading a guide from the folks at the Monterey Bay Aquarium from their website at www.montereybayaquarium.org. I love scrod because this species of fish is widely available and its flakes mingle beautifully with the vegetables in this high-flavored, quick curry dish. Choose fresh store-cut vegetable blends with cruciferous vegetables like broccoli and cauliflower mixed with peppers and snow peas.

Yield:	Prep time:	Cooking time:
4 servings	about 1 minute	about 4 minutes

Ingredients:

Olive oil cooking spray (such as Pam)

16 ounces boneless, skinless scrod filet, cut into 4 equal portions

Salt and freshly ground black pepper

4 cups store-cut vegetables (look for stir-fry blends)

2 cups frozen brown rice and vegetable mix (such as Birds Eye Steamfresh)

2 tablespoons yellow curry powder

3 cups water

2 1/2 tablespoons arrowroot

Method:

1. *Spray* a large nonstick skillet with cooking spray and place over medium-high heat. *Season* the fish filets with salt and pepper, place in the skillet, and *cook* until one side is nicely browned, about 1 minute. Flip the fish and repeat. Remove the fish and set aside on a plate. *Add* the vegetables in the skillet and *cook* until softened, about another minute. Remove the vegetables to a bowl with the rice and set aside.

2. *Whisk* the curry powder, water, and arrowroot together in a bowl. Put the mixture in the skillet and *cook* over high heat until it simmers and is thick, about 30 seconds. *Add* the vegetable and rice mixture to the skillet and toss to coat with the sauce. Spoon evenly onto four plates, top with the roasted fish, and serve.

Tip:

• Add 1/4 cup fresh cilantro to each dish for a fresh flavor at 1 extra calorie per serving.

Per serving:

199 calories, 1.5g fat (0.6g sat), 48.5mg cholesterol, 72mg sodium, 21.5g carbohydrate, 4g fiber, 24g protein

Nutrient content claims:

Reduced calorie / Low fat / Low saturated fat / No sugar added / Good source of fiber / High protein / Trans fat free / Gluten free / Low sodium

Recommended ready-made version:
Wegman's Gazpacho
Calories: 80 / Fat: 4.5g

BEFORE

860 | 51
calories | fat (grams)

AFTER

199 | 1.5
calories | fat (grams)

whisk & simmer

season

add & cook

spray

cook

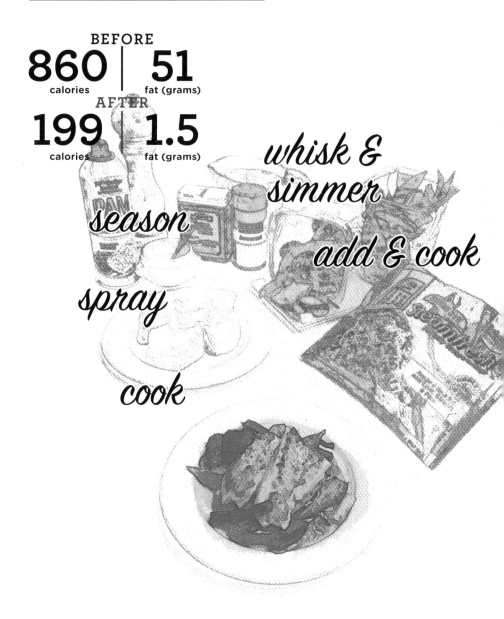

ROASTED SCROD WITH VEGETABLE CURRY

SALMON TERIYAKI WITH GRAPEFRUIT AND FENNEL

C | 210
F | 7.5g

I GET EXCITED when I can get huge flavor returns with little time invested. This fresh dish touches all your taste buds, while you barely touch a knife! This is a great dish to serve for any lunch or dinner, period.

Yield:	Prep time:	Cooking time:
4 servings	about 1 minute	about 5 minutes

Ingredients:

2 cups store-prepared grapefruit sections plus their juice, cut into bite-sized pieces

1 teaspoon no-added-salt-or-sugar wasabi powder (such as Eden)

3 cups fennel bulb, sliced ¼ inch thick across the grain
Olive oil cooking spray (such as Pam)

12 ounces boneless, skinless sockeye, Chinook, or king salmon filet, cut into 4 portions
Salt and freshly ground black pepper

6 tablespoons reduced-sodium sugar-free teriyaki sauce (such as Seal Sama)

Method:

1. Place the grapefruit in a mixing bowl with its juice, *mix* in the wasabi and fennel, and set aside.

2. *Spray* a large nonstick skillet with cooking spray and place over medium-high heat. Season both sides of the salmon portions with salt and pepper and, once the skillet is extremely hot, place the fish in the skillet. *Cook* the salmon until it is beginning to blacken on one side, about 1 minute, then flip and cook until almost blackened on the other side.

3. Turn off the heat and *add* the teriyaki sauce, turning the salmon filets to *coat* well, and let stand in the skillet until just warmed through, about 2 minutes. Divide the grapefruit and fennel salad among 4 bowls and place a piece of salmon over each salad. Spoon any residual sauce from the skillet over the top and serve.

Tips:

- If it appears that all the sauce is going to evaporate during cooking, add a splash of water to the skillet.
- Use wild salmon when possible—it's much healthier!

Per serving:

210 calories, 7.5g fat (1.275g sat), 25.5mg cholesterol, 523.5mg sodium, 15.5g carbohydrate, 3.5g fiber, 18.8g protein

Nutrient content claims:
Reduced calorie / Reduced fat / No added sugar / High protein / Trans fat free /
Good source of fiber

Recommended ready-made version:
Lean Cuisine Salmon with Basil
Calories: 250 / Fat: 2.5g

BEFORE

610 | 13
calories | fat (grams)

AFTER

210 | 7.5
calories | fat (grams)

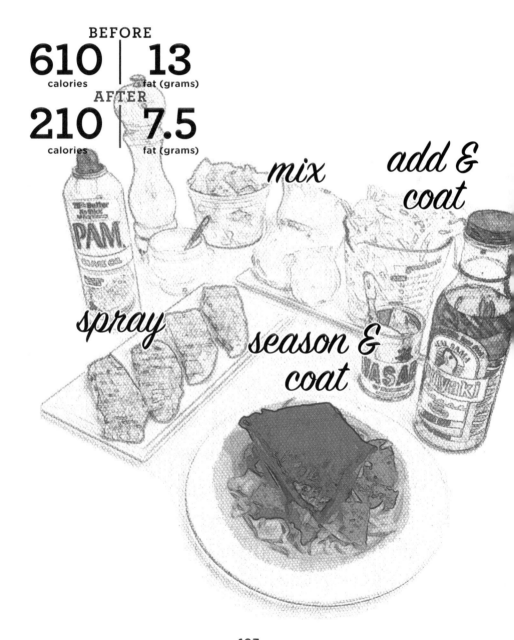

mix

add & coat

spray

season & coat

SALMON TERIYAKI WITH GRAPEFRUIT AND FENNEL

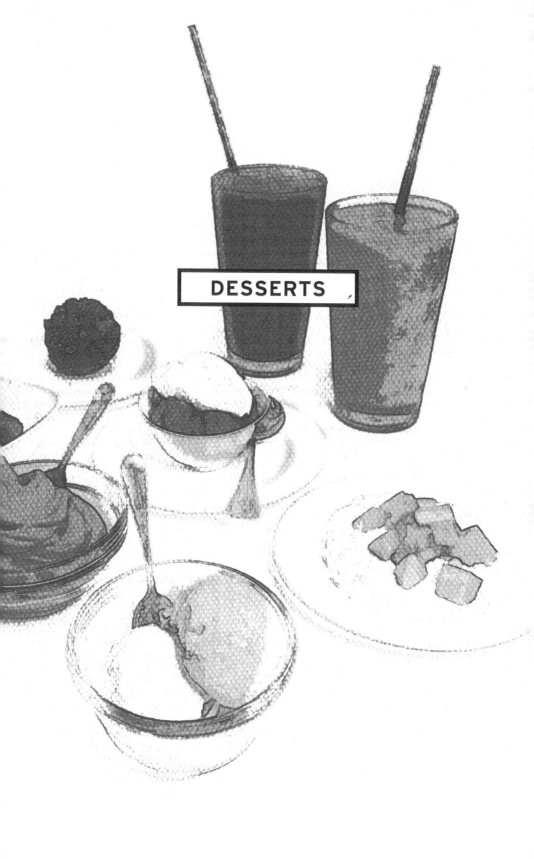

DESSERTS

HIGH-PROTEIN "RICE" PUDDING WITH PAPAYA

C | 83
F | 1g

THIS RECIPE IS extremely easy and a great way to fool your taste buds into thinking they are in serious dessert town. The papaya contains an enzyme that aides in the digestion of protein, so it's the perfect match here.

Yield:	Prep time:	Cooking time:
4 servings	about 5 minutes	about 2 minutes

Ingredients:

1½ cups nonfat cottage cheese (such as Friendship)
2 sugar-free reduced-calorie vanilla pudding cups (such as Jell-O)
2 tablespoons liquid sugar-free vanilla creamer (such as Coffee-mate)
4 packets monk fruit extract (such as Monk Fruit In The Raw)
   Pinch of salt
1 cup fresh diced papaya

Method:

1. Empty the cottage cheese into a mixing bowl, *cover* it with cold water, and *stir* gently to separate the curds from the creamy part. *Scoop* out the curds with a small colander and *strain* out residual water.

2. In another bowl, *combine* the pudding cups, creamer, monk fruit extract, and salt and mix well. Add the curds to the pudding mixture and gently mix together. Spoon the pudding into four small bowls, *top* each dish with ¼ cup of papaya, and serve.

Tip:

• There are many different flavors of reduced-calorie pudding cups out there, so you can use this recipe and make a variety of flavors!

Per serving:

81 calories, 1g fat (0g sat), 3mg cholesterol, 248mg sodium, 13g carbohydrate, 0.5g fiber, 5.5g protein

Nutrient content claims:

Reduced calorie / Low fat / Saturated fat free / Low cholesterol / No added sugar / Gluten free

---

Recommended ready-made version:
Jell-O Sugar-Free Rice Pudding Crème Brûlée
Calories: 70 / Fat: 2g

BEFORE

230 calories | **4.5** fat (grams)

AFTER

83 calories | **1** fat (grams)

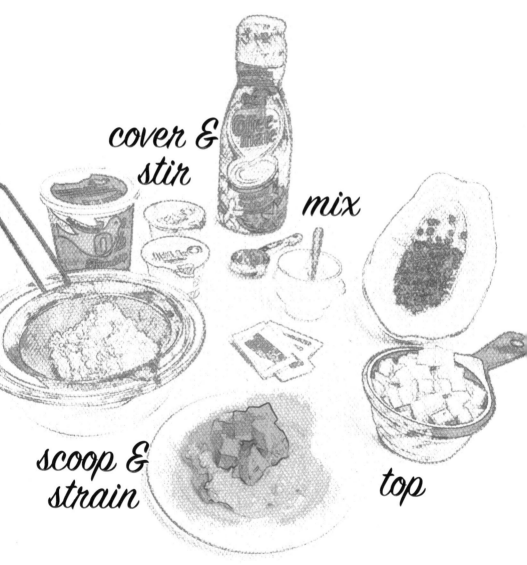

*cover &
stir*

mix

*scoop &
strain*

top

HIGH-PROTEIN "RICE" PUDDING WITH PAPAYA

INSTANT VANILLA FROZEN YOGURT IN A BLENDER

C | 86
F | 1g

YOU JUST CANNOT give up ice cream, ever. I use Greek yogurt and vanilla pudding in this recipe to get a great creamy soft-serve texture. Using the monk fruit extract keeps it sweet while adding no processed sugar or artificial sweeteners. Plus, by adding the 2% Greek yogurt, I get a shot of valuable probiotics as well as protein.

Yield:	Prep/Processing time:	Freezing time:
4 servings	about 5 minutes	6 hours

Ingredients:

3	sugar-free, low-fat vanilla pudding cups (such as Jell-O)
6	ounces 2% Greek yogurt (such as Fage Total 2%)
1/2	cup unsweetened vanilla almond milk (such as Silk)
2	teaspoons all-natural or pure vanilla extract
8	packets monk fruit extract (such as Monk Fruit In The Raw)
	Pinch of salt

Method:

1. *Freeze* the pudding and yogurt separately in ice cube trays until very hard, at least 6 hours.

2. *Pour* the almond milk, vanilla, monk fruit extract, and salt into a blender and *blend* until mixed, about 30 seconds. *Add* the frozen pudding and yogurt cubes and *blend* on high until smooth, pushing down occasionally with the wand or other device provided with your blender. Serve immediately.

Tips:

- Put the almond milk in the blender container in the freezer before you make this recipe. This will help combat the heat generated during blending and keep your frozen dessert nicely frozen.
- If you're planning on keeping this in the freezer for a while, add 1/2 teaspoon xanthan gum to the almond milk and blend on low for 1 minute; this will help prevent crystallization.

Per serving:

86 calories, 1g fat (0g sat), 2.25mg cholesterol, 162mg sodium, 12g carbohydrate, 1.275g fiber, 4.41g protein

Nutrient content claims:

Reduced calorie / Low fat / Saturated fat free / No added sugar / Trans fat free / Gluten free / Low cholesterol

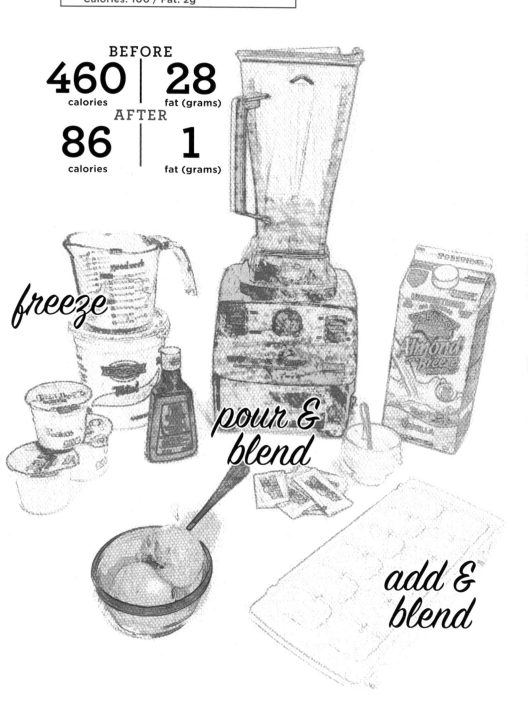

BEFORE

460 calories | **28** fat (grams)

AFTER

86 calories | **1** fat (grams)

freeze

pour & blend

add & blend

INSTANT CHOCOLATE
SOFT-SERVE IN A JUICER

C | 82
F | 0.5g

ITALIAN ICE is enjoyed all over America at street fairs and other events. Italian ice is made like sorbet—that is to say, it's frozen flavored sugar water. I use frozen bananas (a little green is better) in this recipe to get a great creamy soft-serve texture, and with the addition of xanthan gum and natural sweeteners, I've eliminated all processed sugar.

Yield:	Prep time:	Processing time:
Four 4-ounce servings	2 minutes	3 minutes (6 hours freezing time)

Ingredients:

3   packets monk fruit extract (such as Monk Fruit In The Raw)

½   teaspoon xanthan gum (such as Bob's Red Mill)

2   tablespoons water

7   teaspoons unsweetened cocoa powder (such as Hershey's Special Dark)

1   tablespoon organic fat-free milk powder (such as Organic Valley)

2   cups sliced banana (slightly underripe)

     pinch salt

Method:

1. *Mix* the monk fruit extract and xanthan gum in a small mixing bowl and set aside. *Pour* the water into a medium mixing bowl, *add* the cocoa, salt, and milk powder, then slowly *sprinkle* the monk fruit–gum mixture over the water while *whisking* vigorously. *Toss* with the bananas, place in an airtight bag, and *freeze* until solid, about 6 hours. This mixture can keep up to a month.

2. *Process* the banana mixture in a vegetable juicer and serve.

Tips:

• If you don't have a vegetable juicer, you can make this in a high-powered blender. First freeze the bananas, then simply put all the ingredients except for the bananas in the blender and blend. Then add the frozen bananas and blend until smooth while pushing the mixture down into the blade with the wand or bat that came with your blender.

• Put the blender container in the freezer before you make this recipe. This will help combat the heat generated during blending and keep your frozen dessert nicely frozen.

Per serving:

82 calories, 0.5g fat (0g sat), 0mg cholesterol, 50mg sodium, 20.5g carbohydrate, 3.4g fiber, 2.2g protein

BEFORE

188.5
calories

12.5
fat (grams)

AFTER

82
calories

0.5
fat (grams)

process

add, sprinkle, & whisk

mix

toss & freeze

INSTANT CHOCOLATE SOFT-SERVE IN A JUICER

FROZEN STRAWBERRY SHAKE

C | 81
F | 1g

THIS REFRESHING SMOOTHIE is great because it will keep you nice and full for a long time, and with no added sugar and fat free, it won't drag you down at all.

Yield:	Prep time:	Cooking time:
Four 16-ounce dessert smoothies	about 3 minutes	about 2 minutes

Ingredients:

4	cups water
16	packets monk fruit extract (such as Monk Fruit In The Raw)
1/4	cup sugar-free vanilla creamer (such as Coffee-Mate)
3	tablespoons fat-free milk powder
2	heaping cups unsweetened frozen strawberries
3	tablespoons instant sugar-free vanilla pudding mix (such as Jell-O)
1	cup crushed or small cubed ice

Method:

1. *Add* the water to the blender with the monk fruit extract, creamer, milk powder, and half the strawberries and *blend* on high until smooth, about 30 seconds. Turn off the blender, *add* the pudding mix, and *blend* on medium until the mixture has thickened. Turn off the blender.

2. *Add* the ice and the remaining strawberries to the blender and *blend* on high until smooth but still frozen and icy. Pour evenly into four pint-sized glasses and serve.

Per serving:
81 calories, 1g fat (0 g sat), 1.25mg cholesterol, 262.5mg sodium, 1.25g carbohydrate, 1.5g fiber, 2.75g protein

Nutrient content claims:
Reduced calorie / Low fat / Saturated fat free / Cholesterol free / No added sugar / Gluten free

---

Recommended ready-made version:
Pure Protein Banana Strawberry Shake
Calories: 160 / Fat: 1g

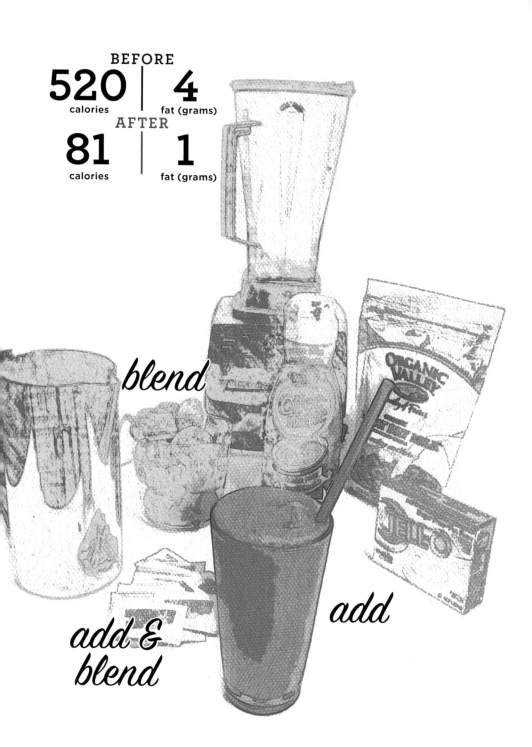

BEFORE
520 | **4**
calories | fat (grams)

AFTER
81 | **1**
calories | fat (grams)

blend

add

*add &
blend*

FROZEN DARK
CHOCOLATE SHAKE

C | 91
F | 1.5g

THIS SMOOTHIE can be made in a flash, and who doesn't love a chocolate shake for dessert? Additionally, when the fat and calories in this smoothie are compared to the fat and calories of a traditional chocolate shake…well, I'll let the numbers do the talking.

Yield:	Prep time:	Blend time:
Four 16-ounce dessert smoothies	about 2 minutes	about 3 minutes

Ingredients:

- 1½ cups cold water
- ½ cup plus 2 tablespoons dark unsweetened cocoa powder (such as Hershey's Special Dark)
- 3 tablespoons organic fat-free milk powder
- 1¼ boxes (5 tablespoons) instant sugar-free chocolate pudding mix (such as Jell-O)
- 12 packets monk fruit extract (such as Monk Fruit In The Raw)
- Pinch of salt
- 6½ cups crushed or small cubes of ice

Method:

1. Place the water, cocoa, monk fruit extract, and milk powder in a blender and *blend* until smooth, about 30 seconds. *Add* the pudding mix and *blend* on low until very thick, about 30 seconds. Shut off the blender.

2. Add the ice to the blender, turn on high, and *blend* until smooth but still cold enough to remain thick, 30 to 45 seconds. Pour into four pint glasses and serve.

Per serving:

91 calories, 1.5g fat (0g sat), 1.5mg cholesterol, 582.5mg sodium, 20.75g carbohydrate, 5g fiber, 4.75 g protein

Nutrient content claims:

Reduced calorie / Low fat / Saturated fat free / Cholesterol free / High fiber / No added sugar / Trans fat free / Gluten free

> *Recommended Ready Made Version:*
> Atkins Advantage Chocolate Royal Shake
> Calories: 160 / Fat: 10g

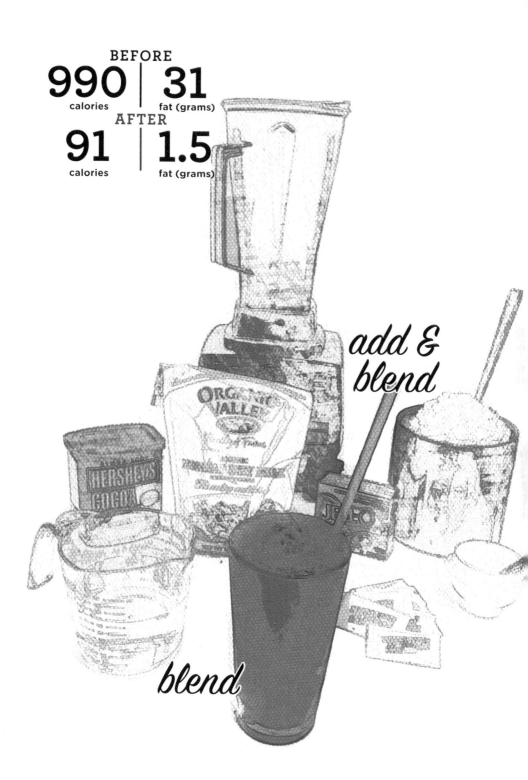

BEFORE

990 calories | 31 fat (grams)

AFTER

91 calories | 1.5 fat (grams)

add & blend

blend

ROCCO'S QUICK-FILL CHOCOLATE-STRAWBERRY BAR
C | 82
F | 0.5g

THIS IS A REAL TREAT—not only to eat, but also because it's made so quickly you won't believe it! This bar is gluten free and has no added sugar and it's practically fat free! Don't worry too much about the bar shape—sometimes I just wrap the whole mess into a few balls and simply tear off pieces as I need them.

Yield:	Prep time:	Cooking time:
4 servings	about 5 minutes	about 5 minutes

Ingredients:

Olive oil cooking spray (such as Pam)

2½ tablespoons coconut nectar

½ cup freeze-dried strawberries, broken into small pieces

2 unsalted brown rice cakes (such as Lundberg)

3 tablespoons dark unsweetened cocoa powder (such as Hershey's Special Dark)

Pinch of salt

4 packets monk fruit extract (such as Monk Fruit In The Raw)

Method:

1. Lay four pieces of plastic wrap (about 10 inches wide each) onto a clean work surface and *spray* with cooking spray.

2. *Combine* the coconut nectar and strawberries in a microwave-safe bowl and *cook* until the coconut nectar starts to simmer, about 30 seconds. Put the remaining ingredients in a small mixing bowl, *mix* well, then place four even piles into each piece of plastic wrap.

3. Fold the corners of one of the plastic wrap pieces to meet in the middle and then press the mixture into a ball. Repeat with remaining mixture.

Tip:

• This is a great base you can use to personalize your own bar. Try adding these to the recipe:

  • 1 tablespoon toasted pumpkin seeds for an additional 10 calories
  • ½ tablespoon mini sugar-free chocolate chips for an additional 7.25 calories

Per serving:

82 calories, 0.5g fat (0g sat), 0mg cholesterol, 61.75mg sodium, 19.8g carbohydrate, 2.6g fiber, 1.3g protein

Reduced calorie / Low fat / Saturated fat free / Cholesterol free / Low sodium / No added sugar / Trans fat free / Gluten free / Good source of fiber

Recommended ready-made version:
Kellogg's Special K Chocolatey Strawberry Cereal Bars
Calories: 90 / Fat: 2g

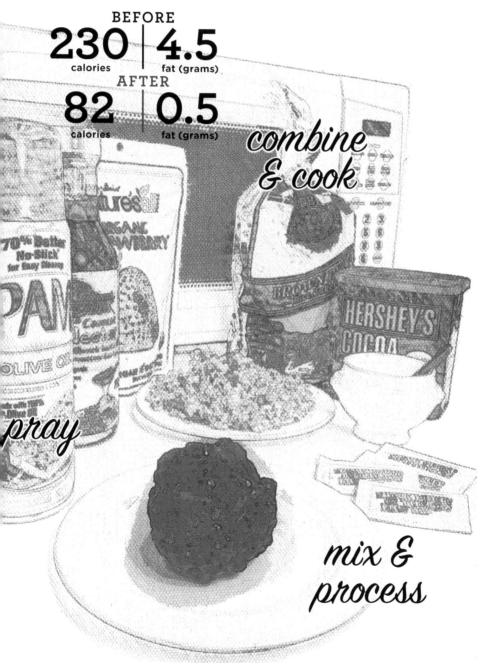

BEFORE

230 calories | **4.5** fat (grams)

AFTER

82 calories | **0.5** fat (grams)

combine & cook

pray

mix & process

ROCCO'S QUICK-FILL CHOCOLATE-STRAWBERRY BAR

FRESH RASPBERRIES WITH
SUGAR-FREE VANILLA CREAM

C | 83
F | 1.5g

SOMETIMES YOU JUST need a touch of whipped cream to make your fresh summer berries extra special.

Yield:	Prep time:	Cooking time:
4 desserts	about 1 minute	about 3 minutes

Ingredients:

1 6-ounce sugar-free reduced-calorie vanilla pudding cup (such as Jell-O)
1 6-ounce container plain Greek-style yogurt (such as Fage 0%)
3 tablespoons sugar-free liquid vanilla creamer (such as Coffee-mate)
3 packets monk fruit extract (such as Monk Fruit In The Raw)
2 cups fresh raspberries, washed

Method:

1. Gently *whisk* the pudding, yogurt, creamer, and monk fruit together in a mixing bowl until well combined.

2. Evenly *distribute* the berries in four bowls and top evenly with whipped cream.

Tips:

- Sprinkle 2 tablespoons freeze-dried raspberries (or other berry) over each of the dishes for a great crispy crunch for an additional 13 calories.
- Try a little fresh mint mixed in with the berries for an added refreshing sensation for 0 calories.

Per serving:

83 calories, 1.5g fat (0g sat), 0mg cholesterol, 59.25mg sodium, 13.5g carbohydrate, 4g fiber, 5.5g protein

Nutrient content claims:

Reduced calorie / Low fat / Saturated fat free / Cholesterol free / Low sodium / Good source of fiber / No added sugar / Trans fat free / Gluten free

Recommended ready-made version:
Activia Parfait Crunch Mixed Berry Yogurt
Calories: 220 / Fat: 3g

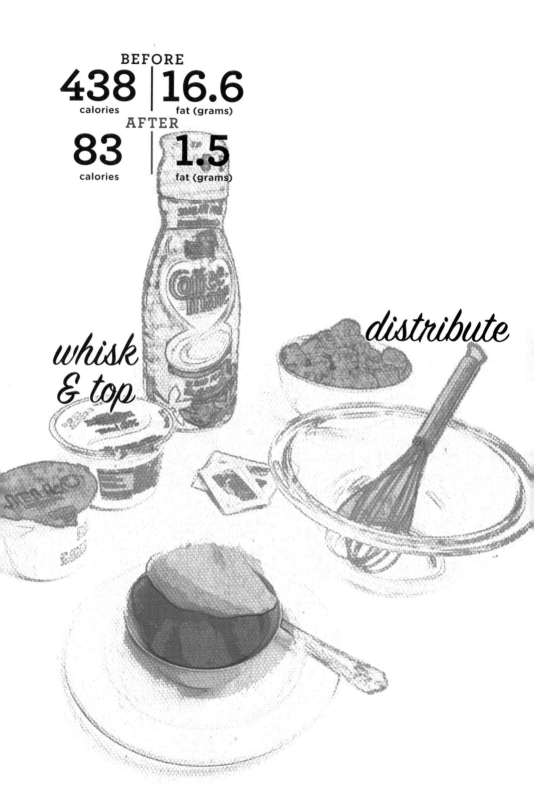

BEFORE

438 calories | **16.6** fat (grams)

AFTER

83 calories | **1.5** fat (grams)

whisk & top

distribute

FRESH RASPBERRIES WITH SUGAR-FREE VANILLA CREAM

FRESH STRAWBERRIES WITH SUGAR-FREE CHOCOLATE SAUCE

C | 49
F | 0.5g

THIS IS A KILLER sauce for all sorts of things: use it for chocolate milk, ice cream toppings, or drizzled over any fruit you like for a super-low-calorie sweet tooth suppressor!

Yield:	Prep time:	Blend time:
Four 1-ounce servings	about 3 minutes	about 1 minute

Ingredients:

- ½ cup water
- Pinch of salt
- 1 tablespoon light agave nectar
- 4 packets monk fruit extract (such as Monk Fruit In The Raw)
- 3 tablespoons plus 1 teaspoon dark unsweetened cocoa powder (such as Hershey's Special Dark)
- ¼ plus ⅛ teaspoon xanthan gum (see Tip below)
- 2 cups fresh halved strawberries, cut into bite-sized pieces

Method:

1. Add the water, salt, agave, monk fruit extract, and cocoa powder to a blender and *blend* on low until everything is incorporated, about 1 minute. *Sprinkle* the xanthan gum while blender is still running and *blend* until thick, about another minute, and turn off the blender.

2. *Distribute* ½ cup of strawberries each into 4 small bowls and evenly pour the sauce over each dish.

Tip:

- The amount of xanthan gum may vary depending on the brand and how it was stored.

Per serving:

49 calories, 0.5g fat (0g sat), 0mg cholesterol, 54.5mg sodium, 12.5g carbohydrate, 3.5g fiber, 1.25g protein

Nutrient content claims:

Reduced calorie / Low fat / Saturated fat free / Cholesterol free / No added sugar / Good source of fiber / Trans fat free / Gluten free / Low sodium

---

Recommended ready-made version:
Strawberries with Smuckers Sugar Free Chocolate Sauce
Calories: 45 / Fat: 0g

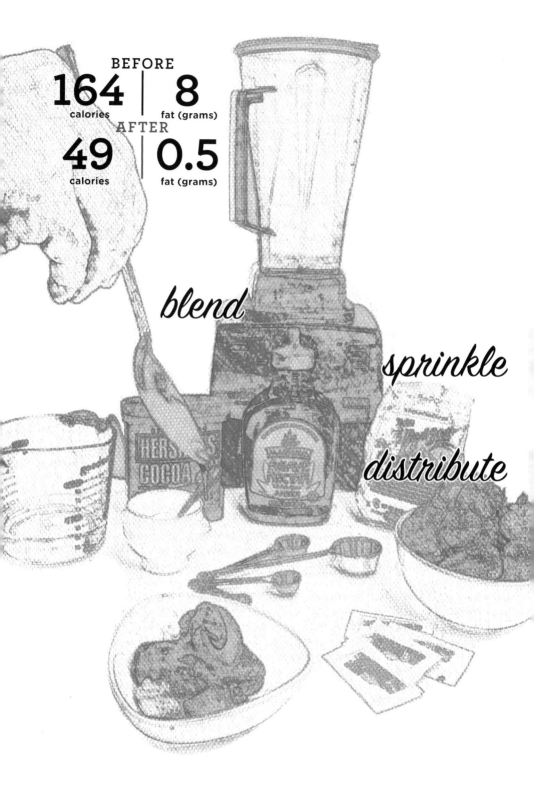

blend

sprinkle

distribute

FRESH STRAWBERRIES WITH SUGAR-FREE CHOCOLATE SAUCE

TROUBLESHOOTING TIPS

The Pound a Day Diet is fast and effective—if you just want to drop a few pounds before that high school reunion or other special event, it may only take you five days. Anyone can stick to something for just five days. Even so, you may encounter stumbling blocks from one day to the next. Below are the answers to a few questions that might arise while you're on the plan.

I just don't like fish. Is there something I can eat instead?

If you don't like fish, of course, don't eat it. If a diet "forces" you to eat something you dislike, you won't stay with that diet for very long. In place of fish, you can substitute chicken, turkey, or another lean protein. Just be sure to look up the calorie count so you'll know you're within the necessary calorie range.

Is it permissible to use condiments such as ketchup, chili sauce, and mustard on my meat or fish?

Definitely. Use these condiments in moderation to enhance the flavors of your foods. Chili sauce, mustard sauce, and other hot spices provide an additional benefit worth reemphasizing. These spices have been shown to increase the body's metabolic rate, an acceleration that can help with fat burning.

I'm a vegetarian. Can I still go on your diet?

The diet is very flexible in this regard. For example, if you're a lacto-ovo vegetarian, you typically limit your animal protein to dairy products and eggs; therefore, substitute these proteins for fish, chicken, and meat. And if you're a semivegetarian who avoids red meat but eats fish or chicken, you can easily follow the diet. Even a vegan, who avoids all animal protein, can follow this diet by substituting legumes for fish, chicken, and meat. You should still be able to lose an appreciable amount of weight.

I'm allergic to wheat. How can I adjust the diet to accommodate my food allergy?

You're not alone if you've found out that you should leave wheat and foods containing it off your plate. Wheat allergies affect one in every 300 people. With a wheat allergy, you must avoid foods that contain gluten, a form of protein found not only in wheat but also in barley and rye. An acceptable substitute for you is rice. If your sensitivity to wheat is less severe, oatmeal and oat bran may be tolerable as well.

Check with your health food store for information on wheat-free and gluten-free products (some foods labeled wheat free are not necessarily gluten free). As you plan your nutrition, focus on the foods you can eat, rather than what you can't eat. Work with your physician, or a registered dietitian, to plan healthy wheat-free meals.

The Skinny on Weight Loss Success

I am a painter and a musician and I recently finished a year-and-a-half tour in Europe during which I put on a lot of weight. As you can imagine, backstage you eat a lot of junk: catered food, candy bars, very irregular eating. I have a tendency to gain weight quickly if I don't eat healthfully. I'm not the kind of woman who can eat whatever she wants and still look fabulous. I've always managed to maintain a certain level of fitness but I completely got off track while on tour.

My aim was to get back into shape—I was getting married and wanted to fit into my dress! I started Rocco's diet at 138 pounds. By the sixth day I had lost six pounds, and about two months later, I was 120 pounds.

The best thing about this diet is that you don't have to think about food anymore. I've tried other diets and felt like I was eating very little food. This time I felt good, like a normal person. It was a completely different experience. You eat five times a day, so you don't have time to be hungry. I never starved on this diet. I was never, ever hungry at all.

All your preconceived ideas of dieting—of not eating, of skipping meals—don't work. With this diet, you're eating, and you're losing weight. You're eating things you'd eat when you're not on a diet, but they're still low fat and low calorie.

With Rocco, you have the mix of a nutrition expert and a chef. His program teaches you to have respect for what you are eating, and to respect your body. Once you've done his diet you won't want to go back to unhealthy eating.

—Chloe

PART THREE

PHASE 2 MAINTENANCE AND MORE

CHAPTER 7

At Your Goal

What to Do Next

CONGRATULATIONS—you've reached your goal weight!

Maybe it happened on day seven of the diet, or day fourteen, or day twenty-eight, or maybe you're well on track to hit a healthy weight in the foreseeable future by putting the insights in this book into action.

You've stepped on a scale and realized that thanks to healthy, low-calorie eating and regular physical activity, and thanks to the power of Diet Booster Foods and creating a calorie deficit, you're now at or closer to a normal, healthy body weight.

Now what?

Now that you've lost weight and are looking great, it's time to think about maintaining your new shape. Unless you have a long-term plan in place for doing so, you will join the ever-swelling ranks of unsuccessful dieters, people who have regained their lost weight. It's an unfortunate fact that most dieters will regain as much as two-thirds of their lost pounds within a year. Don't be among them. Please don't be among them!

As you've already discovered, you can shed as many as five pounds, or more, in a fairly short time. You've trimmed down to a smaller dress or pants size, and your body feels great. Your entire outlook has changed.

The low-calorie phase of the diet is over and it's time to shift into a delicious food lifestyle you can savor for the rest of your life.

First, let's look at what estimated weight range you should shoot to stay at over the long term.

YOUR TARGET ZONE

If you're a woman, your goal is to slenderize down to a waist size of thirty-five inches or less, and stay there. If you're a man, your waist size should be forty inches or less. You can use a simple tape-measure test to determine this.

But the most widely used index to determine optimal body weight and health is the BMI, or body mass index.

According to the National Institutes of Health, the BMI is a good measure of overweight and obesity. It's calculated from your height and weight, and it's an estimate of body fat and a good gauge of your risk for diseases that can come with more body fat. The higher your BMI number, the greater your risk of diseases like heart disease, high blood pressure, type 2 diabetes, gallstones, breathing problems, and certain cancers. Although the BMI can be used for most adults, it's an estimate, not a perfect measure. It may overestimate body fat in athletes and others who have a muscular build, and it may underestimate body fat in older people and others who have lost muscle.

The BMI score means:

BMI

Underweight	Below 18.5
Normal	18.5 to 24.9, THIS IS YOUR TARGET!
Overweight	25.0 to 29.9
Obese	30.0 and above

Here's a chart to help you calculate your BMI:

How Smoking Hot Is Your Body?

Normal	Smoking Hot Body! You've Nailed Your Weight
Overweight	Let's Get Hot Again
Obese	We've Got Some Serious Work to Do
Extremely Obese	Get Me Out of Here! Let's Get You to a Doctor, Fast

	NORMAL					OVERWEIGHT						OBESE				
BMI	19	20	21	22	23	24	25	26	27	28	29	30	31	32	33	34	35
Height (inches)						**Body Weight (pounds)**											
58	91	96	100	105	110	115	119	124	129	134	138	143	148	153	158	162	167
59	94	99	104	109	114	119	124	128	133	138	143	148	153	158	163	168	173
60	97	102	107	112	118	123	128	133	138	143	148	153	158	163	168	174	179
61	100	106	111	116	122	127	132	137	143	148	153	158	164	169	174	180	185
62	104	109	115	120	126	131	136	142	147	153	158	164	169	175	180	186	191
63	107	113	118	124	130	135	141	146	152	158	163	169	175	180	186	191	197
64	110	116	122	128	134	140	145	151	157	163	169	174	180	186	192	197	204
65	114	120	126	132	138	144	150	156	162	168	174	180	186	192	198	204	210
66	118	124	130	136	142	148	155	161	167	173	179	186	192	198	204	210	216
67	121	127	134	140	146	153	159	166	172	178	185	191	198	204	211	217	223
68	125	131	138	144	151	158	164	171	177	184	190	197	203	210	216	223	230
69	128	135	142	149	155	162	169	176	182	189	196	203	209	216	223	230	236
70	132	139	146	153	160	167	174	181	188	195	202	209	216	222	229	236	243
71	136	143	150	157	165	172	179	186	193	200	208	215	222	229	236	243	250
72	140	147	154	162	169	177	184	191	199	206	213	221	228	235	242	250	258
73	144	151	159	166	174	182	189	197	204	212	219	227	235	242	250	257	265
74	148	155	163	171	179	186	194	202	210	218	225	233	241	249	256	264	272
75	152	160	168	176	184	192	200	208	216	224	232	240	248	256	264	272	279
76	156	164	172	180	189	197	205	213	221	230	238	246	254	263	271	279	287

(continued)

	OBESE								EXTREMELY OBESE										
BMI	36	37	38	39	40	41	42	43	44	45	46	47	48	49	50	51	52	53	54
Height (inches)									**Body Weight (pounds)**										
58	172	177	181	186	191	196	201	205	210	215	220	224	229	234	239	244	248	253	258
59	178	183	188	193	198	203	208	212	217	222	227	232	237	242	247	252	257	262	267
60	184	189	194	199	204	209	215	220	225	230	235	240	245	250	255	261	266	271	276
61	190	195	201	206	211	217	222	227	232	238	243	248	254	259	264	269	275	280	285
62	196	202	207	213	218	224	229	235	240	246	251	256	262	267	273	278	284	289	295
63	203	208	214	220	225	231	237	242	248	254	259	265	270	278	282	287	293	299	304
64	209	215	221	227	232	238	244	250	256	262	267	273	279	285	291	296	302	308	314
65	216	222	228	234	240	246	252	258	264	270	276	282	288	294	300	306	312	318	324
66	223	229	235	241	247	253	260	266	272	278	284	291	297	303	309	315	322	328	334
67	230	236	242	249	255	261	268	274	280	287	293	299	306	312	319	325	331	338	344
68	236	243	249	256	262	269	276	282	289	295	302	308	315	322	328	335	341	348	354
69	243	250	257	263	270	277	284	291	297	304	311	318	324	331	338	345	351	358	365
70	250	257	264	271	278	285	292	299	306	313	320	327	334	341	348	355	362	369	376
71	257	265	272	279	286	293	301	308	315	322	329	338	343	351	358	365	372	379	386
72	265	272	279	287	294	302	309	316	324	331	338	346	353	361	368	375	383	390	397
73	272	280	288	295	302	310	318	325	333	340	348	355	363	371	378	386	393	401	408
74	280	287	295	303	311	319	326	334	342	350	358	365	373	381	389	396	404	412	420
75	287	295	303	311	319	327	335	343	351	359	367	375	383	391	399	407	415	423	431
76	295	304	312	320	328	336	344	353	361	369	377	385	394	402	410	418	426	435	443

Source: Adapted from Clinical Guidelines on the Identification, Evaluation, and Treatment of Overweight and Obesity in Adults: The Evidence Report.

Once you get to a healthy weight, here are estimates of how many calories you should be taking in:

YOUR MAGIC WEIGHT NUMBER

This Is How Many Calories You Should Be Taking in per Day Once You're at a Healthy Weight, to Stay at a Healthy Weight

If You Are Female*	Sedentary	Moderately Active	Active
19–30	1,800–2,000	2,000–2,200	2,400
31–50	1,800	2,000	2,200
51+	1,600	1,800	2,000–2,200
Male			
19–30	2,400–2,600	2,600–2,800	3,000
31–50	2,200–2,400	2,400–2,600	2,800–3,000
51+	2,000–2,200	2,200–2,400	2,400–2,800

* Not pregnant or breastfeeding.

Note: Estimated numbers of calories needed to maintain calorie balance, rounded to nearest 200 calories. An individual's calorie needs may be higher or lower than these average estimates.

Source: Dietary Guidelines for Americans

I don't think you need to get calorie obsessed (though it probably works for some people!) but it really pays to be *calorie aware*. To keep the weight off successfully, it's very important to avoid an all-or-nothing mentality. Of course you're going to overeat occasionally. Of course you're going to have some less healthy food and have high-calorie days now and then. It's OK! Forgive yourself! What matters most is that the *overall pattern* of your eating over the course of days and weeks stays healthy and in line with the Mediterranean diet pattern and in line with your calorie range in the chart above.

To keep the weight off over the long term, remember the lessons of Phase 1: Focus on an overall carb-corrected, calorie-corrected healthy eating pattern.

Here's a traffic-light formula to guide your food lifestyle, which is a key to your lasting weight loss and health:

The Master List of Foods You Should Base Your Diet On—to Lose Weight and Keep It Off

Green-Light Foods:	*Enjoy as often as you like!*
Yellow-Light Foods:	*Enjoy often; keep an eye on portion sizes and calories.*
Red-Light Foods:	*Eat rarely or not at all.*

GREEN-LIGHT FOODS

Enjoy as often as you like!

Fruits and Vegetables

Almost all fruits and vegetables can be considered green-light super-foods—as long as you:

- Eat a wide variety of them—think of "eating the rainbow" of bright colors through the week as a way of varying the produce you enjoy.

- Prepare them in healthy ways, like steaming, baking, or flash-frying (more on that later!).

- Add salt very sparingly, or not at all.

- Avoid eating them fried very often.

- Eat them as close to their original whole state as possible (sorry, most potato and veggie chips don't count, although I make a killer kale chip).

Some experts have a grudge against potatoes and recommend you eat them only sparingly, as they score high on the glycemic index of foods that are likely to spike your blood sugar and perhaps, over time, contribute to weight gain. Personally I've got nothing against having spuds from time to time as long as they're eaten as part of an overall diet rich in lots of different kinds of veggies and fruits.

Remember, the big news is that all fruits and veggies are good for you one way or another. They help control your appetite, fill you up, and satisfy your hunger better than other foods. Many of them are nutrient dense: they are chock-full of fiber and a host of other nutrients that help you lose weight and stay healthy, especially versus processed foods. According to the 2010 Dietary Guidelines for Americans, there are at least three huge reasons to load up on the fruits and veggies:

1. *When prepared without added fats or sugars, they're relatively low in calories. Eating them instead of higher-calorie foods can help adults and children achieve and maintain a healthy weight.*

2. *They're major contributors of a number of nutrients you may not be getting enough of, like folate, magnesium, potassium, dietary fiber, and vitamins A, C, and K. Several of these are of concern for the general public, like dietary fiber and potassium; or for a specific group, like folate for women who may become pregnant.*

3. *They're associated with reduced risk of many chronic diseases. Specifically, moderate evidence indicates that intake of at least two and a half cups of vegetables and fruits per day is associated with a reduced risk of cardiovascular disease, including heart attack and stroke. Some vegetables and fruits may be protective against certain types of cancer.*

Be sure to include choices like these in your overall rotation:

- *Red and orange vegetables:* tomatoes, red peppers, carrots, sweet potatoes and yams (excellent sources of beta-carotene and vitamin C, by the way, and don't add extra sugar, they're naturally sweet!), squash, and pumpkin.

- *Dark-green vegetables:* broccoli; spinach; romaine; and collard, turnip, and mustard greens.

- **Beans and peas (legumes):** kidney beans, lentils, garbanzos (aka chickpeas), and pinto beans. These are superb sources of fiber, protein, slow carbs, and other nutrients.

- **Fruits:** apples, apricots, bananas, dates, grapes, oranges, grapefruits, mangoes, melons, peaches, pineapples, raisins, strawberries, blueberries, and tangerines.

- **Other produce:** like cauliflower, zucchini, green beans and green peas, onions, and corn.

- **Ultra-low-calorie fruits and veggies:** include celery, cucumbers, oranges, tangerines, grapefruits, apples, zucchini, squash, sea veggies like kelp, asparagus, apricots, watermelon, tomatoes, strawberries, leafy greens, arugula, red bell peppers, turnips, Brussels sprouts, beets, and cauliflower.

I prefer to buy seasonal, organic, and local fruits and veggies as often as I can, but canned and frozen produce count, too.

YELLOW-LIGHT FOODS

Enjoy often, but keep an eye on portion sizes and calories.

- **Whole grains:** oatmeal, brown rice, barley, buckwheat groats or kasha, millet, and quinoa. Oatmeal is my go-to fill-me-up food for a quick snack or breakfast.

- **Eggs, lean cuts of meat and poultry:** but use them more as a garnish than a big main dish. Follow the example of Italy, where I've noticed that a 2-ounce meat portion is typical. Don't think that's too small—it's actually the right size! Select only lean; trim away visible fat; broil, roast, or poach; remove skin from poultry. To err on the side of caution, limit your egg yolk intake to no more than four per week; two egg whites have the same protein content as 1 ounce of meat.

- **Nuts and seeds:** almonds, walnuts, flaxseeds, brazil nuts, cashews, pecans, pine nuts, pistachios, and peanuts. Most are good sources of protein and good fats, but eat them unsalted and keep an extra-careful eye on portion sizes and nutrition label calorie information, as the calories can add up quickly.

- **Low-fat and no-fat dairy products:** if you choose to enjoy them.

- **Healthy oils:** like olive oil and canola oil.

- **Fish:** a great protein source, and fatty fish like salmon are a superb source of heart-healthy omega-3 fatty acids. If you're concerned about mercury, PCBs, and sustainability, here's a handy chart from the Environmental Defense Fund for you to refer to when making fish choices in the supermarket. The fish in the left-hand column are best, especially the ones with the heart symbol.

Popular Seafood: Best and Worst Choices

FISH	ECO-BEST	ECO-OK	ECO-WORST
Salmon	• Canned salmon♥ • Wild salmon from Alaska♥	• Wild salmon from Washington▲ • Wild salmon from California • Wild salmon from Oregon	• Farmed or Atlantic salmon▲
Shrimp	• Pink shrimp from Oregon • Spot prawns from Canada	• Brown shrimp • Farmed shrimp from US • Northern shrimp from US and Canada • Spot prawns from US • White shrimp • Wild shrimp from US	• Blue shrimp • Chinese white shrimp • Giant tiger prawns • Imported shrimp and prawns

FISH	ECO-BEST	ECO-OK	ECO-WORST
Tilapia	• Tilapia from US	• Tilapia from Latin America	• Tilapia from Asia
Trout	• Farmed rainbow trout♥		
Tuna	• Albacore from US or Canada♥ • Yellowfin from US Atlantic caught by troll/pole♥	• Canned light tuna • Canned white/albacore ▲ • Imported bigeye/yellowfin caught by troll/pole ▲	• Albacore tuna (imported longline) ▲ • Bluefin tuna ▲ • Imported bigeye/yellowfin tuna caught by longline ▲

♥ = Indicates fish high in heart-healthy omega-3 fatty acids and low in environmental contaminants.

▲ = Indicates fish high in mercury or PCBs.

"Eco-best" means harvested by an environmentally sustainable method.

Source: Environmental Defense Fund

Extra notes on fish from the Dietary Guidelines for Americans:

- An intake of 8 or more ounces per week of a variety of seafood is recommended for adults. Seafood contributes a range of nutrients, notably the omega-3 fatty acids EPA and DHA. Moderate evidence shows that consumption of about 8 ounces per week of a variety of seafood, which provide an average consumption of 250 milligrams per day of EPA and DHA, is associated with reduced cardiac deaths among individuals with and without preexisting cardiovascular disease. Thus, this recommendation contributes to the prevention of heart disease. The recommendation is to consume seafood for the total package of benefits it provides, including its EPA and DHA content.

- Seafood varieties commonly consumed in the United States that are higher in EPA and DHA and lower in methylmercury include salmon, anchovies, herring, sardines, Pacific oysters, trout, and Atlantic and Pacific mackerel (not king mackerel, which is high in methylmercury).

- In addition to the health benefits for the general public, the nutritional value of seafood is of particular importance during fetal growth and development, as well as in early infancy and childhood. Moderate evidence indicates that intake of omega-3 fatty acids, in particular DHA, from at least 8 ounces of seafood per week for women who are pregnant or breastfeeding is associated with improved infant health outcomes, such as visual and cognitive development. Therefore, it is recommended that women who are pregnant or breastfeeding consume at least 8 and up to 12 ounces of a variety of seafood per week, from choices that are lower in methyl mercury. Obstetricians and pediatricians should provide guidance to women who are pregnant or breastfeeding to help them make healthy food choices that include seafood.

RED-LIGHT FOODS

Consume rarely or not at all.

- Foods high in saturated fat, added sugars, and sodium.

- Sweetened beverages like soda and fruit drinks. Instead of fruit juice, go for the whole fruit.

- Highly processed snacks and foods.

- *Note:* Sweet snacks and treats are fine, but eat them only occasionally, and in small portions.

SHOCKER ALERT: WHAT SERVING SIZES REALLY SHOULD LOOK LIKE

Did you know that a proper serving of meat is only the size of a deck of cards?

Or that a serving of a leafy veggie like spinach should be as big as a baseball?

Or that a serving of pasta should look like half a baseball?

It's time to rebalance your view of serving sizes! Here's the scoop:

FOOD	SERVING	LOOKS LIKE
Chopped vegetables	1/2 cup	1/2 baseball
Raw leafy vegetables	1 cup	1 baseball or fist for average adult
Fresh fruit	1 medium piece	1 baseball
	1/2 cup chopped	1/2 baseball
Dried fruit	1/4 cup	1 golf ball
Pasta, rice, cooked cereal	1/2 cup	1/2 baseball
Red meat, poultry, seafood	3 oz. (boneless cooked weight from 4 oz. raw)	Deck of cards
Dried beans	1/2 cup cooked	1/2 baseball
Nuts	1/3 cup	Level handful for average adult
Cheese	1 1/2 oz.	4 dice or 2 nine-volt batteries

Sources: US Department of Agriculture, AICR.org

SECRETS OF THE WORLD'S GREATEST DIETS

People in many parts of the world enjoy longer, healthier lives and smaller waistlines than we do in America.

In many parts of the Mediterranean, Asia, and elsewhere, the reasons are a more physically active lifestyle and a much healthier everyday dietary pattern.

Some common threads emerge from these dietary patterns, with lessons that can help you lose weight and keep it off:

- They are abundant in unprocessed, whole vegetables and fruits.

- Many emphasize whole grains.

- They include moderate amounts and a variety of foods high in protein—seafood, beans and peas, nuts, seeds, soy products, meat, poultry, and eggs.

- They include only limited amounts of foods high in added sugars.

- Most are low in full-fat milk and milk products.

- However, some include substantial amounts of low-fat milk and milk products. In some patterns, wine is included with meals.

- Compared to typical American diets, these patterns tend to have a high unsaturated-to-saturated fat ratio and a high dietary fiber and potassium content.

- In addition, some are relatively low in sodium compared to current American intake.

- They feature fewer processed foods and more correct portion sizes than typical American diets.

- They are not based on fad diets, gimmicks, denial, or cutting out food groups but on enjoying food in the right amounts and patterns.

Source: Adapted from Dietary Guidelines for Americans

Read the Labels!

I think it's extremely important that you read the nutrition information labels on the backs of food and beverage packages. That should be your starting point.

You've got to know what's in the food; otherwise, you're just guessing. And this plan requires some precise ingredients and some precise elements.

You have to look for things like calories, sodium levels, sugars, fats, fiber, and protein. You should be looking at both ingredients and the nutrition information.

And you've got to pay very close attention to both the serving size and the number of servings in a package. It's pretty complicated, probably more complicated than it needs to be, probably on purpose. But you've got to put in the time to do it.

If you're serious about healthy eating and you want to make sure you're consuming the number of calories you want to consume, you absolutely have to do it. I do it. I've been doing it religiously for about six years.

I don't put a thing in my mouth that I haven't read the nutrition information for, with very few exceptions. I'm on calorieking.com constantly. I'm on it. It's like Facebook for me!

MY DIET JOURNAL

It's also a great idea to keep a diet journal like this one to stay motivated and on track and to pinpoint your setbacks as well as celebrate your triumphs:

Make a pile of blank copies of this page and the next, tape it to your refrigerator or bulletin board, and fill in the details every day:

Goals for the Week

My Food Goals

- I will enjoy a plant-based diet based on whole foods, not processed foods.

- I will power up the fruits, veggies, and whole grains and enjoy lean sources of protein like beans and fish.

- I will dial down the sodium, added sugars, and portion sizes and be extra mindful of calories.

- I will take control by cooking fast and easy at home whenever I can.

My Physical Activity Goals

- I will do at least forty-five minutes of moderate-intensity physical activity most days of the week, like brisk walking, all at once or divided into sessions of at least ten minutes.

My Weight Loss Goals

- I will get to a healthy weight and stay there—through healthy eating and physical activity.

- I will enjoy food—regular meals and snacks—and I will focus on the foods I can savor.

- I will not diet anymore. Instead, I will shift to a healthy food and exercise lifestyle based on the principles in this book, and I will enjoy it for the rest of my life!

- After a few weeks and months, I will send my success story to Rocco's Facebook page (facebook.com/RoccoDiSpirito) for the world to see.

Include daily calorie totals when eating Rocco's recipes from *The Pound a Day Diet*:

	Starting Day						*Weigh-In Day*
	MON	TUE	WED	THU	FRI	SAT	SUN
							My weight:
Breakfast							
Lunch							
Dinner							
Snacks							
Physical activity (type and total minutes)							
How did I feel today, and what can I be thankful for, about food and life?							

The Skinny on Weight Loss Success

I'm a fifty-five-year-old guy, I work at a desk all day, and I was looking to lose about five to seven pounds, to get from the "overweight" zone to the "normal weight" category. Rocco's plan worked out great, and I steadily lost almost a pound a day over the course of a week.

I call this the "eat all day" diet, because that's what you do! It was a beautiful, delicious rhythm of healthy food in controlled-calorie portions, and I never felt deprived at all.

The first thing in the morning every day, I had a chocolate protein smoothie. Then a grapefruit for breakfast. An hour or two later I'd have a midmorning snack like an egg-white omelet or sweet potato chips. For lunch, I savored meals like a chopped salad with grilled chicken and carrot ginger dressing, or gazpacho with grilled shrimp, which is unbelievably good. Then a midday snack, and a fantastic dinner!

The amazing thing is that the meals are all filling, so I felt satisfied and happy, not weak or dizzy or starving like I have on other diets. I went from 192 to 186 in a week, and I loved every minute. The diet works because it's based on good science, and the success you experience feeds on itself.

—Jason

MEGA-SECRET FOR KEEPING THE WEIGHT OFF FOR GOOD: FROM NOW ON, EAT LIKE A MEDITERRANEAN MAMA

It's time for you to eat like a Mediterranean mama. You heard me!

The Mediterranean dietary pattern is the basis of my maintenance plan.

Ahhh…Italy.

Italian mamas' cooking. Olives picked fresh from the fields that feel like velvet on your tongue. Homemade pasta cooked with fresh peppers, herbs, and veggies grown in the backyard. And every meal saturated in laughter, conversation, and love.

On my last trip to Italy, I ate like a king for three weeks, and I lost ten pounds. It always happens to me when I go there. I savor the most magnificent food on earth, I have three or more hearty meals a day, and I lose weight.

That's because in many parts of Italy, they still enjoy the centuries-old dietary pattern that modern science is increasingly hailing as the closest thing to a perfect pattern for weight control, longevity, and overall health: the Ultimate Diet Pattern of the Mediterranean-style diet, based on the traditional diets of Italy, Spain, Greece, and other Mediterranean food utopias.

If you want to be slim and healthy, eat like a native Italian.

In Italy, the lifestyle contributes to the overall healthiness of the population. It's not just the food; it's the lifestyle. Italians eat local foods as a matter of pride and for practicality. What makes sense for them is to eat what grows around them.

When you ask about an Amalfi coast lemon and somebody is from Sorrento, only sixteen kilometers away, they'll say, "Oh, we don't have those here." Those lemons are grown in Amalfi—it's only a ten-minute drive!

When you consider that Americans habitually ship foods five thousand or eight thousand miles, the Italian regional food sensibility is very strong. Italians almost all participate in the growing of some kind of food or livestock, and they almost all participate in this 365-day-a-year system of cultivating, producing, harvesting, and preserving the food that will sustain them the whole year. I was in Italy cooking a dish that required asparagus, and they said, "There is no asparagus this time of year; you won't find any." If it isn't fresh, they don't eat it, period, and rarely will they eat food that's been frozen.

Without question, part of what contributes to the success of the Italians' diet is their lifestyle. It's a lifestyle that's focused on regional products, regional cooking, and regional tradition, tried and tested over hundreds if not thousands of years. It's also a very interlaced social system where everyone has everyone's back. It's very difficult to go hungry in Italy.

I think that in America, there's less of the socializing that goes with eating. In Italy it all works in one big beautiful system. If your next meal doesn't come from money you've earned, then it will come from your friends and family. There's less stress about where your next meal is coming from, and less stressful eating than there is in the United States.

People don't feel isolated in Italy. They understand that there's always going to be someone to take care of them, or they're going to be taking care of someone else, and there's always going to be some food to eat. They don't eat every meal like it's their last meal. They're not filling the void that comes with loneliness and depression and anxiety with the thrill of eating in desperation to get stuffed.

Great food causes thrills—a chemical reaction to great flavor and the pleasure that comes with that and the chemicals that are released in the brain. Italian food does that.

The eating experience is such a rich one. Everyone stops working for meals; there are a lot of people at the table; there's a lot of movement and talking, activity and laughter. Eating is not just putting food in your mouth; it's also the social experience that comes with it.

I always advise people to talk while you eat—you'll eat less!

If you look at what Italians eat, you'll see that it just so happens that their portions are half what ours are in America. A portion of meat is between two and four ounces. When's the last time you saw someone order a four-ounce steak in America?

Here is a Mediterranean Diet Pyramid that I love so much that I've stuck it on my refrigerator to remind myself of how beautiful the diet is and how easy it is to enjoy.

I've incorporated the principles of this lifestyle into my program, and I live by them daily.

This lifestyle is not a strict set of rules to obsess over, but a beautiful pattern of eating to savor with your family for the rest of your life.

This is literally the way you should eat for the rest of your life!

Note on portion sizes: Because foods in the bottom section of the pyramid may be eaten in larger amounts and more frequently, portion sizes and frequency of consumption decline in the pyramid's upper sections.

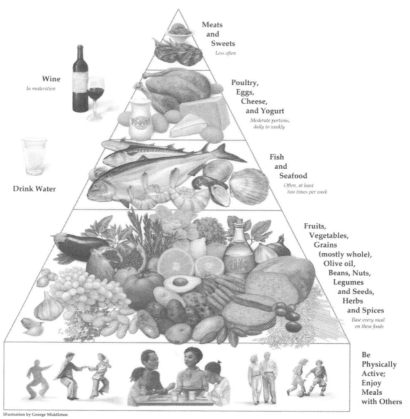

The Mediterranean Diet Pyramid

Meats
and
Sweets
Less often

Wine
In moderation

Poultry,
Eggs,
Cheese,
and Yogurt
*Moderate portions,
daily to weekly*

Drink Water

Fish
and
Seafood
*Often, at least
two times per week*

Fruits,
Vegetables,
Grains
(mostly whole),
Olive oil,
Beans, Nuts,
Legumes
and Seeds,
Herbs
and Spices
*Base every meal
on these foods*

Be
Physically
Active;
Enjoy
Meals
with Others

Illustration by George Middleton

© 2009 Oldways Preservation and Exchange Trust   www.oldwayspt.org

EIGHT SUPER-FAST TIPS TO START LOSING WEIGHT RIGHT NOW

by Eating Like a Mediterranean

1. **Eat lots of vegetables.** From a simple plate of sliced fresh tomatoes drizzled with olive oil and crumbled feta cheese to stunning salads, garlicky greens, fragrant soups and stews, healthy pizzas, and oven-roasted medleys, vegetables are vitally important to the fresh tastes and delicious flavors of the Mediterranean diet.

2. **Change the way you think about meat.** If you eat meat, have smaller amounts—small strips of sirloin in a vegetable sauté, or a dish of pasta garnished with diced prosciutto.

3. **Always eat breakfast.** Start your day with fiber-rich foods such as fruit and whole grains to keep you pleasantly full for hours. Layer granola, yogurt, and fruit, or mash half an avocado with a fork and spread it on a slice of whole-grain toast.

4. **Eat seafood twice a week.** Fish such as tuna, herring, salmon, and sardines are rich in omega-3 fatty acids, and shellfish including mussels, oysters, and clams have similar benefits for brain and heart health.

5. **Cook a vegetarian meal one night a week.** Build meals around beans, whole grains, and vegetables, and heighten the flavor with fragrant herbs and spices. Down the road, try two nights per week.

6. **Use good fats.** Include sources of healthy fats in daily meals, especially extra virgin olive oil, nuts, peanuts, sunflower seeds, olives, and avocados.

7. **Enjoy some dairy products.** Eat Greek or plain yogurt, and try small amounts of a variety of cheeses.

8. **For dessert, eat fresh fruit.** Choose from a wide range of delicious fresh fruits—from fresh figs and oranges to pomegranates, grapes, and apples. Instead of daily ice cream or cookies, save sweets for a special treat or celebration.

Source: Oldways Preservation Trust

I've got more great news for you—believe it or not, there is a magic pill that will supercharge the weight control effects of calorie correction, carb correction, Diet Booster Foods, and the Mediterranean diet.

Like to know what it is?

Hint: It involves short pants...and sneakers.

The Skinny on Weight Loss Success

I started at 200 pounds, which is my "red flag" weight, above which I don't want to go. It was good timing that I started Rocco's diet, because I was right at that point, the summer was coming, and I wanted to look good. I was on Rocco's plan for three weeks, and I actually got lower than my goal weight of 185. And I've actually been able to maintain the weight loss. I'm now at 182. I'm six feet tall and I just turned fifty-four years old.

The program worked really well. It felt great to lose the pounds. But what was more important to me than the pounds were the inches. Before I started the diet, my waist was at thirty-eight inches, and it ended up at thirty-five. I went from a forty-four-inch chest to about a forty.

The food was great. I liked the fact that the portions were manageable. I thought they were going to be a little bit slight, but they were just right.

Now that I'm off the diet, I'm following the food principles—smaller and more frequent meals—and exercising at an appropriate heart rate. I'm able to do all the principles on my own.

Losing the weight was motivational. Now I want to keep it off. I feel good about my health, and I feel really good about the way I look. I want to keep it up!

I am the lowest weight I've been in twenty years. People are saying things to me like "What are you doing? You look really fit!" Or "You look the best you've ever looked, you look a lot younger!" At the gym, someone told me someone else was checking me out and asking "Who's that guy with the nice body?" I haven't heard that in twenty years.

That's motivating!

—Chris

CHAPTER 8

Ten Minutes to Fitness

The Magic Pill for Fast, Healthy Weight Loss

WANT TO LOSE some serious weight?

Guess what—only two brisk ten-minute walks per day can give you a huge jump-start toward your goal.

And to close the deal, it may take only three or four brisk fifteen-minute walks per day, combined with a delicious calorie-corrected eating pattern.

How simple is that?

Hey, what are we waiting for? *Let's go already!*

I have discovered a weight loss miracle.

It works miracles for me and it will work miracles for you, too.

What if I told you I'd found a magic pill that blasts fat off your body?

Its benefits are endorsed by the world's greatest experts on diet and weight loss.

Not only does it work with the food you eat to melt the pounds away and keep them off; it makes you feel great, it protects you against a wide range of illnesses, and best of all, you can get it totally free of charge.

It's not a medicine you take in a capsule form.

It's something you put on your feet.

They're called sneakers, and the miracle they deliver is exercise and physical activity. When you put them into action, they will totally change your life for the better.

I will make a true confession to you.

When I was at my fattest, I didn't exercise.

I was working around the clock in my restaurant, and that was it.

Normally, all that working in the kitchen would burn off a lot of calories, but since I was overeating all that great food and I wasn't making the time to do any regular, structured physical activity, it helped pack the pounds onto my belly.

But today, it's a whole different story.

I'm in the greatest shape of my life. I've discovered that exercise is an absolute joy, and a powerful tool to help you lose weight and stay lean.

Do you know what the biggest secret is about getting in shape?

The secret is this: Once you do it, *you feel fantastic!*

These days, I do cardio work like cycling four to six times per week at 18 to 19 miles per hour for forty minutes or more, plus resistance training at least three times a week. I also build regular physical activity into my daily mind-set and life rhythms. I'm lucky to live in Manhattan so that I can walk everywhere, and all that pounding the pavement really helps keep me in shape. I fly up and down stairs whenever I can, and whenever I'm presented with a choice between doing things the lazy way (taking a taxi a few blocks) and doing things the fun, physical way (like a brisk walk to my destination), I'll chose to get moving.

If you want to lose weight and keep it off, you've got to exercise.

There's no way around it. To lose weight, you've got to create a calorie deficit over days and weeks, and exercise (the structured kind) and physical activity (which is exercise plus all the day-to-day stuff that can also burn off calories) is a critical piece of that deficit, combined with healthy eating. You just can't expect to lose weight and keep it off successfully if you don't exercise. The surprising news is that for most people, physical activity alone isn't enough to lose much weight. If you want to move into a more successful healthy lifestyle where you can sometimes indulge in your favorite foods and not worry about it, you've got to burn off surplus calories.

The great news is that when combined with healthy, calorie-corrected eating patterns, physical activity can both help you lose weight and provide a measure of insurance that it won't come back on, if you stick with it and build it into your lifestyle as a pleasurable activity you love and look forward to.

Twenty-one minutes a day of moderate-intensity physical activity like brisk walking is all you need to put this miracle to work. That's all you need to start getting healthy, especially if you combine it with calorie-corrected eating.

To crank up the fat-burning effects of exercise into high gear, work up to thirty-four minutes a day of moderate-intensity physical activity. That can be just two brisk seventeen-minute walks.

You **can** do it!

Exercise is a great way to maintain weight loss and make up for occasional "cheating." You're going to cheat every once in a while; you're going to go off your healthy eating pattern. There are going to be periods when you weigh more and periods when you weigh less. The way to work out the peaks and valleys and keep the line smooth is through exercise. Not to mention that you have to put on more muscle mass in order for your body to burn calories at a higher rate.

I may never grace the cover of a men's fitness magazine. But I have learned that when I work out regularly I can take off weight pretty fast and eat almost as much of anything as I want, within reason, and the pounds stay off. That's enough motivation for me to keep exercising.

Most people think you have to work out for thirty to sixty minutes straight to get fit. For a lot of us, this is unrealistic—and a recommendation that only about 15 percent of Americans comply with. Most people complain that they "don't have time" for that much exercise.

Here's more good news: Recently, a new wave of research has confirmed that you can achieve the same calorie burn with short, intense workouts that you do with long, steady workouts. I recently switched from two-hour bike rides in the morning to really fast thirty-minute rides. And I can already see a difference. I can see a difference in endurance, in fat burn; I can see little bits of my abs peeking out faster than usual.

Shorter exercise sessions spread through the day can deliver results equal to or better than long gym sessions. According to research published in the *Journal of Applied Physiology*, people who take a break in the middle of their workout burn more fat than those who do a single session. Other studies have found that three ten-minute bouts of exercise a day are as effective for weight loss as one thirty-minute session. "Doing split sessions means you can work harder as you're less likely to run out of steam, plus it keeps your metabolic rate and improved insulin resistance peaking, in turn, reducing appetite," reported exercise physiologist and dietitian Joanne Turner in the March 1, 2011, edition of *Good Health*.

Did You Know?

- According to the Centers for Disease Control and Prevention, 60 percent of Americans are not meeting the recommended levels of physical activity.

- Fully 16 percent of Americans are not active at all. Overall, women tend to be less active than men, and older people are less likely to get regular physical activity than younger individuals.

- 10.8 percent of all premature deaths in the United States are now related to too little exercise, according to a study quoted in a July 18, 2012, *New York Times* article.

- Over 31 percent of the world's adults, or about 1.5 billion people, are almost completely sedentary, meaning that they do not meet the minimum recommendation of 150 minutes of walking or other moderate activity per week, or about 20 minutes a day. "I don't think most people really understand that not exercising," even if someone is otherwise healthy, "appears to be just as unhealthy" as smoking or being obese, lead researcher Dr. I-Min Lee of the Harvard School of Public Health told the *Times*.

A few years ago, the US government convened an all-star "dream team" panel of the greatest experts on health and asked them to review the evidence on the health benefits of physical activity for a report called the *Physical Activity Guidelines for Americans*. And they revealed some striking findings on how physical activity can help you melt the pounds away and supercharge your health. They found moderate-to-strong evidence that for adults, regular physical activity is associated with a wide range of fantastic benefits, including weight control.

THE THREE FAT-BLASTING EFFECTS OF REGULAR PHYSICAL ACTIVITY

Regular physical activity can help you:

1. *Lose weight, especially when combined with reduced calorie intake.*

2. *Reduce abdominal fat—and preserve muscle while you're losing weight.*

3. *Maintain healthy weight after weight loss and prevent weight gain.*

THE TWENTY-FIVE BONUS EFFECTS THAT SUPERCHARGE YOUR HEALTH

Regular physical activity can also:

1. *Strengthen your heart muscle, which improves your heart's ability to pump blood to your lungs and throughout your body. As a result, more blood flows to your muscles, and oxygen levels in your blood rise. Capillaries, your body's tiny blood vessels, also widen. This allows them to deliver more oxygen to your body and carry away waste products.*

2. *Give you more energy throughout your busy day.*

3. *Lower your risk of early death.*

4. *Lower your risk of coronary heart disease.*

5. *Lower your risk of stroke.*

6. *Lower your risk of high blood pressure.*

7. *Lower your risk of adverse blood lipid profile and raise your HDL (good) cholesterol levels.*

8. *Help your body manage blood sugar and insulin levels, which lowers your risk of type 2 diabetes.*

9. *Lower your risk of metabolic syndrome.*

10. *Lower your risk of colon, breast, endometrial, and lung cancer.*

11. *Improve your cardiorespiratory and muscular fitness.*

12. *Prevent falls.*

13. *Reduce depression; help you beat the blues.*

14. *Help you relax and cope better with stress.*

15. *Build your confidence.*

16. *Improve your cognitive function (for older adults).*

17. *Improve your functional health (for older adults).*

18. *Lower your risk of hip fracture.*

19. *Lower your risk of cancer.*

20. *Increase your bone density and slow bone loss.*

21. *Improve the quality of your sleep and allow you to fall asleep more quickly and sleep more soundly.*

22. *Strengthen your lungs and help them work more efficiently.*

23. *Tone and strengthen your muscles and build your stamina.*

24. *Keep your joints in good condition.*

25. *Improve your balance.*

It's amazing that you can achieve all this by doing one incredibly easy, simple, and free thing: put your sneakers on and walk briskly for forty-five minutes a day. If it's raining, watch TV and briskly march in place for forty-five minutes—or for twenty-two minutes twice a day, maybe once in the morning and once at night. It's that simple!

In Phase 2 of **The Pound a Day Diet,** you should be performing a minimum of twenty minutes a day of moderate-intensity exercise, like brisk walking, and work up to a regular sixty to ninety minutes a day of moderate-to-intense exercise, on most days of the week, for the rest your active life.

To trigger substantial health benefits, you need at least twenty-one minutes a day of moderate exercise—like two brisk ten-minute walks (hey, I'm rounding).

An average of at least 150 minutes (2 hours and 30 minutes) a week, or 21 minutes a day, of moderate-intensity aerobic exercise like brisk walking delivers major health benefits, including lower risk of premature death, coronary heart disease, stroke, hypertension, type 2 diabetes, and depression.

Aerobic activity should be performed in chunks of at least ten minutes, and for best results it should be spread through the week.

To trigger weight control benefits, you need at least forty-three minutes a day of moderate exercise—like two brisk twenty-two-minute walks.

An average of at least 300 minutes (5 hours) a week, or 43 minutes a day, of moderate-intensity aerobic exercise, like brisk walking, delivers major health benefits and triggers weight control benefits as well (especially when combined with healthier eating), including lower risk of colon and breast cancer and *prevention of unhealthy weight gain.*

To trigger weight loss benefits, you need sixty to ninety minutes a day of moderate exercise.

An average of sixty to ninety minutes a day of moderate-intensity aerobic exercise on most, and preferably all, days of the week can trigger the above health benefits, *plus weight loss benefits*, especially when combined with healthier eating.

Whether you're exercising twenty minutes a day or ninety minutes a day, remember the following:

The ten-minute rule: Aerobic activity should be performed in chunks of at least ten minutes, and for best results it should be spread through the week. Aerobic exercise should preferably be spread throughout the week. Research studies consistently show that exercise performed on at least three days a week produces health benefits. Spreading physical activity across at least three days a week may help reduce the risk of injury and avoid excessive fatigue.

You should also do muscle-strengthening activities that are moderate or vigorous intensity and involve all major muscle groups on two or more days a week, as these activities provide additional health benefits. Muscle-strengthening activity is physical activity, including exercise, that increases skeletal muscle strength, power, endurance, and mass. It includes strength training, resistance training, and muscular strength and endurance exercises. Muscle-strengthening activities include lifting weights, push-ups, and sit-ups. Choose activities that work all the different parts of the body—the legs, hips, back, chest, stomach, shoulders, and arms.

GET RESULTS

The great news if you're as pressed for time as I am: You can cut all the above time estimates in half and get the same benefits if you do vigorous-intensity exercise instead of moderate-intensity exercise. Next, I'll show you some examples of how to do this.

These examples from the *Physical Activity Guidelines for Americans* (PAGA) research show how you can reach target fitness goals by doing moderate-intensity or vigorous-intensity exercise or a combination of both.

GET BIG HEALTH BENEFITS

Ways to get the equivalent of an average of 150 minutes (2 hours and 30 minutes) per week, or 21 minutes per day, of moderate-intensity aerobic exercise a week plus muscle-strengthening activities:

- Thirty minutes of brisk walking (moderate intensity) on five days, and exercising with resistance bands (muscle strengthening) on two days; or,

- Twenty-five minutes of running (vigorous intensity) on three days, and lifting weights (muscle strengthening) on two days; or,

- Thirty minutes of brisk walking on two days, sixty minutes of social dancing (moderate intensity) on one evening, thirty minutes of mowing the lawn (moderate intensity) on one afternoon, and heavy gardening (muscle strengthening) on two days; or,

- Thirty minutes of an aerobic dance class (vigorous intensity) on one morning, thirty minutes of running (vigorous intensity) on one day, thirty minutes of brisk walking (moderate intensity) on one day, and calisthenics such as sit-ups and push-ups (muscle strengthening) on three days; or,

- Thirty minutes of biking to and from work (moderate intensity) on three days, playing softball for sixty minutes (moderate intensity) on one day, and using weight machines (muscle strengthening) on two days; or,

- Forty-five minutes of doubles tennis (moderate intensity) on two days, lifting weights after work (muscle strengthening) on one day, and hiking vigorously for thirty minutes and rock climbing (muscle strengthening) on one day.

GET BIG HEALTH BENEFITS, PLUS A WEIGHT CONTROL EDGE

Ways to get the equivalent of an average of 300 minutes (5 hours) per week, or 43 minutes per day, of moderate-intensity aerobic exercise a week plus muscle-strengthening activities:

- Forty-five minutes of brisk walking every day (which can be broken into more than one walk), and exercising with resistance bands on two or three days, or;

- Forty-five minutes of running on three or four days, and circuit weight training in a gym on two or three days, or;

- Thirty minutes of running on two days, forty-five minutes of brisk walking on one day, forty-five minutes of an aerobics and weights class on one day, ninety minutes of social dancing on one evening, and thirty minutes of mowing the lawn, plus some heavy garden work, on one day, or;

- Ninety minutes of playing soccer on one day, brisk walking for fifteen minutes on three days, and lifting weights on two days, or;

- Forty-five minutes of stationary bicycling on two days, sixty minutes of basketball on two days, and sixty minutes of calisthenics on three days.

Aerobic Physical Activities and Intensity

Moderate Intensity

Moderate-intensity physical activity is aerobic activity that increases a person's heart rate and breathing to some extent. On a scale relative to a person's capacity, moderate-intensity activity is usually a 5 or 6 on a 0-to-10 scale. It causes noticeable increases in breathing and heart rate. A person doing moderate-intensity activity can talk but not sing. Examples of moderate-intensity activity:

- walking briskly (3 miles per hour or faster, but not race-walking)
- water aerobics
- bicycling slower than 10 miles per hour
- tennis (doubles)
- ballroom dancing
- gardening
- canoeing

Vigorous Intensity

Vigorous-intensity physical activity is aerobic activity that greatly increases a person's heart rate and breathing. On a scale relative to a person's capacity, vigorous-intensity activity is usually a 7 or 8 on a 0-to-10 scale. A person doing vigorous-intensity activity can't say more than a few words without stopping for a breath.

With vigorous-intensity activities, you get similar health benefits in half the time it takes with moderate ones. Vigorous-intensity activities make your heart, lungs, and muscles work hard. Examples of vigorous-intensity activities:

- aerobic dance

- jumping rope

- race-walking

- jogging

- running

- soccer

- swimming fast or swimming laps

- riding a bike on hills or riding 10 miles per hour or faster

- tennis (singles)

- heavy gardening (continuous digging or hoeing, with heart rate increases)

- hiking uphill or with a heavy backpack

TYPES OF PHYSICAL ACTIVITY

The four main types of physical activity are aerobic, muscle-strengthening, bone-strengthening, and stretching. Aerobic activity benefits your heart and lungs the most.

Getting weight control and weight loss benefits is largely a function of doing aerobic activities for a certain length of time.

I usually hit all these types of physical activity in the course of a week, and I usually hit my personal target of an average of sixty to ninety minutes of moderate-to-vigorous exercise a day.

- **Aerobic activity** moves your large muscles, such as those in your arms and legs. Running, swimming, walking, biking, dancing, and doing jumping jacks are examples of aerobic activity. Aerobic activity **also is called endurance or cardio activity**. The body's large muscles move in a rhythmic manner for a sustained period. Aerobic activity causes a person's heart to beat faster than usual. The other types of physical activity—muscle-strengthening, bone-strengthening, and stretching—benefit your body in other ways.

- **Muscle-strengthening** activities improve the strength, power, and endurance of your muscles. Doing push-ups and sit-ups, lifting weights, climbing stairs, and digging in the garden are examples of muscle-strengthening activities.

- With **bone-strengthening activities**, your feet, legs, or arms support your body's weight, and your muscles push against your bones. This helps make your bones strong. Running, walking, jumping rope, and lifting weights are examples of bone-strengthening activities. Muscle-strengthening and bone-strengthening activities also can be aerobic. Whether they are depends on whether they make your heart and lungs work harder than usual. For example, running is an aerobic activity and a bone-strengthening activity.

- **Stretching** helps improve your flexibility and your ability to fully move your joints. Touching your toes, doing side stretches, and doing yoga are examples of stretching.

Source: PAGA

HOW TO BLAST OFF THE FAT

There are two ways to lose weight: First, you can choose to eat your usual number of calories but be more active. For example, a 200-pound person who keeps on eating the same number of calories but begins to walk briskly each day for a mile and a half will lose about fourteen pounds in one year. Staying active will also help keep the weight off.

Second, you can eat fewer calories and be more active. This is the best way to lose weight, since you're more likely to be successful by combining a healthful lower-calorie diet with physical activity. For example, a 200-pound person who consumes 250 fewer calories per day and begins to walk briskly each day for a mile and a half will lose about forty pounds in one year.

Most of the energy you burn each day—about three-quarters of it—goes to activities that your body automatically engages in for survival, such as breathing, sleeping, and digesting food. The part of your energy output that **you** control is daily physical activity. Any activity you take part in beyond your body's automatic activities will burn extra calories. Even seated activities, such as using the computer or watching TV, will burn calories—but only a very small number. That's why it's important to make time each day for moderate-to-vigorous physical activity.

Per week, as a general rule of thumb, you need to burn off about 3,500 more calories than you take in, or a deficit of 3,500 calories, to lose one pound. Per day, that means a daily deficit of 500 calories. To lose four pounds a week, you'd need a deficit of 2,000 calories a day (sources: Dietary Guidelines for Americans, National Institutes of Health).

Below are examples of the calorie burn for a 154-pound person. A lighter person will burn fewer calories; a heavier person will burn more. I've also included a sample weekly exercise schedule to help you establish a healthy routine.

Moderate Physical Activity	Calories Burned per Hour
Hiking	370
Light gardening/yard work	330
Dancing	330
Golf (walking and carrying clubs)	330
Bicycling (slower than 10 mph)	290
Walking (3.5 mph)	280
Weight lifting (light workout)	220
Stretching	180

Vigorous Physical Activity	Calories Burned per Hour
Running/jogging	590
Bicycling (faster than 10 mph)	590
Swimming (slow freestyle laps)	510

Aerobics	480
Walking (4.5 mph)	460
Heavy yard work like chopping wood	440
Weight lifting (vigorous workout)	440
Basketball (vigorous)	440

Source: 2005 Dietary Guidelines for Americans Advisory Committee Report

SAMPLE WEEKLY SCHEDULE

SUNDAY	Aerobic		Stretch
MONDAY	Aerobic	Strength	Stretch
TUESDAY	Aerobic		Stretch
WEDNESDAY	Aerobic	Strength	Stretch
THURSDAY	Aerobic		Stretch
FRIDAY	Aerobic	Strength	Stretch
SATURDAY	Aerobic		Stretch

Source: National Institutes of Health

THREE SMART EXTRA MOVES

Other forms of physical activity can also help you burn calories and get healthy. These aren't aerobic activities, but great fun ways to boost your overall physical and mental health, on top of your regular physical activity program:

- **Yoga** can improve flexibility, balance, muscle strength, and relaxation—and a recent study found that regular yoga practice can help minimize weight gain in middle age.

- **Tai chi** is a series of slow movements that shift body weight and flow rhythmically together into one graceful gesture. This gentle, calming practice can help improve flexibility and balance, and it gradually builds muscle strength.

- **Pilates** is a body-conditioning routine that can strengthen and tone muscles as well as increase flexibility.

FITNESS STARTER KIT

A SUPER-EASY POWER-WALKING PROGRAM FOR THE MAINTENANCE PHASE

What's the easiest way to get fit and help your body lose weight?

It's got to be power-walking, otherwise known as brisk walking.

All you need is a pair of comfy shoes, a little spare time, and a smile on your face—that's all it takes.

Brisk walking is a super-simple, enjoyable way to help keep your heart healthy and help achieve a fat-melting calorie deficit. One study showed that regular brisk walking lowers the risk of heart attack by the same amount as more vigorous exercise. Remember that you can break up any activity into shorter periods of at least ten minutes each. For example, if you want to total thirty minutes of activity per day, you could spend ten minutes walking on your lunch break, another ten minutes raking leaves in the backyard, and another ten minutes lifting weights.

Here's a terrific walking program put together by the National Institutes of Health, followed by NIH's sample jogging program.

During each week of the walking program, try to walk briskly at least five days per week. Always start with a five-minute, slower-paced walk to warm up, and end with a five-minute, slower-paced walk to cool down. (Warm-up and cool-down sessions totaling ten minutes are included in the "Total Time per Day" column.) As you walk, check your pulse periodically to see whether you're moving within your target heart rate zone.

WEEK	WARM-UP	TARGET ZONE	COOL-DOWN	TOTAL TIME PER DAY
Week 1	Walk 5 min.	Walk briskly 5 min.	Walk 5 min.	15 min.
Week 2	Walk 5 min.	Walk briskly 7 min.	Walk 5 min.	17 min.
Week 3	Walk 5 min.	Walk briskly 9 min.	Walk 5 min.	19 min.
Week 4	Walk 5 min.	Walk briskly 11 min.	Walk 5 min.	21 min.
Week 5	Walk 5 min.	Walk briskly 13 min.	Walk 5 min.	23 min.

Week 6	Walk 5 min.	Walk briskly 15 min.	Walk 5 min.	25 min.
Week 7	Walk 5 min.	Walk briskly 18 min.	Walk 5 min.	28 min.
Week 8	Walk 5 min.	Walk briskly 20 min.	Walk 5 min.	30 min.
Week 9	Walk 5 min.	Walk briskly 23 min.	Walk 5 min.	33 min.
Week 10	Walk 5 min.	Walk briskly 26 min.	Walk 5 min.	36 min.
Week 11	Walk 5 min.	Walk briskly 28 min.	Walk 5 min.	38 min.
Week 12	Walk 5 min.	Walk briskly 30 min.	Walk 5 min.	40 min.

As you become more fit, try to walk within the upper range of your target zone. Gradually increase your brisk walking time from thirty to sixty minutes, most days of the week. Enjoy the outdoors!

A SAMPLE JOGGING PROGRAM

During each week of the program, try to jog at least five days per week. For your warm-up, walk for five minutes. For your cool-down, walk for three minutes and then stretch for two minutes more. (Warm-up and cool-down sessions totaling ten minutes are included in the "Total Time per Day" column.) As you jog, check your pulse periodically to see whether you're moving within your target heart rate zone. If you're over forty and haven't been active in a while, begin with the walking program. After you complete the walking program, start with Week 3 of the jogging program.

WEEK	WARM-UP	TARGET ZONE	COOL-DOWN	TOTAL TIME PER DAY
Week 1	Walk 5 min., then stretch	Walk 10 min. Try to walk without stopping.	Walk 3 min., stretch 2 min.	20 min.
Week 2	Walk 5 min., then stretch	Walk 5 min., jog 1 min., walk 5 min., jog 1 min.	Walk 3 min., stretch 2 min.	22 min.
Week 3	Walk 5 min., then stretch	Walk 5 min., jog 3 min., walk 5 min., jog 3 min.	Walk 3 min., stretch 2 min.	26 min.

(continued)

WEEK	WARM-UP	TARGET ZONE	COOL-DOWN	TOTAL TIME PER DAY
Week 4	Walk 5 min., then stretch	Walk 4 min., jog 5 min., walk 4 min., jog 5 min.	Walk 3 min., stretch 2 min.	28 min.
Week 5	Walk 5 min., then stretch	Walk 4 min., jog 5 min., walk 4 min., jog 5 min.	Walk 3 min., stretch 2 min.	28 min.
Week 6	Walk 5 min., then stretch	Walk 5 min., jog 6 min., walk 5 min., jog 6 min.	Walk 3 min., stretch 2 min.	32 min.
Week 7	Walk 5 min., then stretch	Walk 4 min., jog 7 min., walk 4 min., jog 7 min.	Walk 3 min., stretch 2 min.	32 min.
Week 8	Walk 5 min., then stretch	Walk 4 min., jog 8 min., walk 4 min., jog 8 min.	Walk 3 min., stretch 2 min.	34 min.
Week 9	Walk 5 min., then stretch	Walk 4 min., jog 9 min., walk 4 min., jog 9 min.	Walk 3 min., stretch 2 min.	36 min.
Week 10	Walk 5 min., then stretch	Walk 4 min., jog 13 min.	Walk 3 min., stretch 2 min.	27 min.
Week 11	Walk 5 min., then stretch	Walk 4 min., jog 15 min.	Walk 3 min., stretch 2 min.	29 min.
Week 12	Walk 5 min., then stretch	Walk 4 min., jog 17 min.	Walk 3 min., stretch 2 min.	31 min.
Week 13	Walk 5 min., then stretch	Walk 2 min., jog slowly 2 min., jog 17 min.	Walk 3 min., stretch 2 min.	31 min.
Week 14	Walk 5 min., then stretch	Walk 1 min., jog slowly 3 min., jog 17 min.	Walk 3 min., stretch 2 min.	31 min.
Week 15	Walk 5 min., then stretch	Jog slowly 3 min., jog 17 min.	Walk 3 min., stretch 2 min.	30 min.

As you become more fit, try to jog within the upper range of your target zone. Gradually, increase your jogging time from twenty to thirty minutes (or up to sixty minutes, if you wish). Keep track of your goals—and keep on enjoying yourself.

TIPS FOR TURNING YOUR BODY INTO A PERPETUAL FAT-MELTING MACHINE

- Use the stairs—both up and down—instead of the elevator. Start with one flight of stairs and gradually build up to more.

- Park a few blocks from the office or store and walk the rest of the way. If you take public transportation, get off a stop or two early and walk a few blocks.

- While working, take frequent activity breaks. Get up and stretch, walk around, and give your muscles and mind a chance to relax.

- Instead of eating that extra snack, take a brisk stroll around the neighborhood or your office building.

- Do housework, gardening, or yard work at a more vigorous pace.

- When you travel, walk around the train station, bus station, or airport rather than sitting and waiting.

- Keep moving while you watch TV. Lift hand weights, do some gentle yoga stretches, or pedal an exercise bike.

- Better yet, turn off the TV and take a brisk walk.

Source: National Institutes of Health

CALORIE-BURNING POWER

Here are more examples of how you can burn off calories, based on two weight levels: 163 pounds, which is roughly the weight of the average American woman, and 190 pounds, which is roughly the weight of the average American man.

Notice how much you can burn off, not just with structured physical exercise, but also with everyday activities!

The big lesson is—walk those extra few blocks with the dog, cook that meal for your family, do those chores a little more often, rake those leaves, walk those five blocks to the grocery store instead of driving—it all adds up!

Calories Burned in Forty-Five Minutes

	163-pound person	190-pound person
Cooking or food preparation	111	129
Cleaning, light, moderate effort	139	162
Gardening	222	259
Pushing stroller with child	139	162
Mowing lawn	305	356
Raking lawn	222	259
Walking, very brisk pace (4 mph)	277	323
Chopping wood	344	401
General aerobics	360	420
Basketball, nongame	333	388
Bicycling, moderate pace (12 to 14 mph)	444	517
General circuit training	444	517
Dancing	250	291
Elliptical trainer	499	582
Hiking, climbing hills (carrying less than a 10-pound load)	394	459
Judo, karate, kickboxing, tae kwon do	555	646
Kickboxing (including Turbo Jam)	560	653
Wii boxing	299	349
Water jogging	444	517
Tennis, singles	444	517
Tae Bo	560	653
Tai chi	222	259
Martial arts	488	569
Swimming laps, freestyle, light-to-moderate effort	388	452
Stationary bike, moderate effort	388	452

Squash	665	776
Spinning	388	452
Soccer, casual	388	452
Slimnastics, Jazzercise	333	388
Running (jogging), in place	444	517

Source: myfitnesspal.com

The Skinny on Weight Loss Success

I've got to tell you, the results from this program are phenomenal! In the first seven days I lost eight pounds. After thirteen days, I lost over twelve pounds. I started at 181 pounds; now I'm just under 169. I'm thirty-six years old, five-nine, with a fairly slim build, and I didn't think I'd lose that much so quickly. I started at a little over 25 body fat percentage and now I'm down to 22.

With this diet you feel like you're eating all day! That's the beauty of it.

Rocco's Pound a Day Diet gives you real food, three full meals and a bunch of snacks, so you gain an increasing awareness of things that work, and things you should be avoiding.

I feel great, I have more energy, I sleep better, my clothes are fitting better, it's all those things you want! The most important thing about this diet is the awareness it creates: what you're eating, how frequently you're eating, how to manage your heart rate, working out, keeping a journal. Before, I'd never really paid attention to any of that stuff. Now that I'm eating really healthy and getting into great shape, it really takes my life to a whole new level.

I love this diet, and I love the fact that on a day-to-day basis, it's just really easy.

—Peter

CHAPTER 9

Cooking for Weight Loss

NOW THAT you're at your goal weight, remember that if you want to control your weight, you have got to cook.

If you want to keep the weight off, I think it's absolutely critical that you learn to cook at home more often.

That's easy for me to say—I've been a professional chef for over twenty years!

But I'm a huge believer in all of us learning to cook at home more often.

I don't care if you heat up tea in a microwave or slap together a peanut butter and jelly sandwich, *you can cook*. Hell, don't get me started, but I think it's healthier to cook at home, more satisfying, and definitely more economical—and that's coming from someone who has been a partner and executive chef in several restaurants.

I'd often rather whip up something delicious and healthy in five minutes than go out to eat. And you can, too. There's no question that you can cook healthy food fast. It does require a slightly different lifestyle, one that calls for some extra planning and just a different approach to things.

Cooking for yourself saves money, it saves time, and it can knock pounds off your waist. The sad truth is that the people who make food commercially, the food manufacturers and the restaurant companies, are not usually looking out for our health. They're not building food that is in our best interest. They're building food that will market well, sell well, make a lot of profit, and last for a long time on the shelf. If you want to put that in your body all the time, that's up to you, but it's usually a bad way to lose weight.

Many of us are two generations away from people who cook. I think that about half the women in America, and at least two-thirds of the men, have either forgotten how to really cook or they never learned in the first place.

I can make you a home chef in five minutes. You just have to try it. I think once people try it one or two times, they typically find it's a lot easier than they expected. For people who absolutely insist they can't cook, I direct them through the process of heating a pan, putting ingredients in a pan, smelling the aromas—and they're hooked.

Cooking for people is the ultimate turn-on. It's the ultimate gesture of kindness and generosity. If you want to tell people that you love them and that they matter in this world, you cook for them. The first thing a mother does when her child is born is to feed it. It's so basic to who we are as beings on this planet, and yet we're so far removed from it.

On the list of things to make you cool, after learning how to play lead guitar and becoming a rock star, I'd say cooking is number two. But the difference is you can learn how to cook very easily. It's not so easy to become Axl Rose. Oh my God. Men who cook? There's nothing sexier to a woman!

When you can cook, you're a different level of person. If you're overweight, you have one more reason to do it. Maybe it's your time to become a foodie, learn how to cook, and lose weight, all at once. I know what you may be thinking.

"Nice idea, Rocco, but forget it. Cook at home? What, are you kidding? Who's got time for that! I'm waaaay too busy. I'll never find the time. Far better to pick up some fast, convenient prepared food and save time."

You may have made this claim to yourself. It's much easier, cheaper, and faster to open a package and eat, right?

Well, think again.

In 2007, an amazing study was published in the *British Food Journal* by researchers from UCLA's Center on Everyday Lives of Families. It was the first academic study to track a small sampling of American families as they made dinner.

Their conclusion: "Surprisingly, dinner didn't get on the table any faster in homes that favored convenience foods. Meals took an average of fifty-two minutes to prepare." Lead researcher Dr. Margaret Beck reported, "People don't spend any less time overall on dinner when they use so-called convenience foods. Families seem to spend a certain amount of time cooking regardless. When commercial items are involved, they just ramp up how elaborate it gets."

It got even more complicated when children are involved, because parents often have to pick up and prepare different "convenience foods" for dinner. Dr. Beck noted, "The kids frequently got entirely separate entrees or separate items from the adults, so that adds to the overall complexity of the meal." Even worse, the kids don't help prepare and serve dinner. Another one of the researchers said, "It makes me sad when I think of people not having this experience. You lose family and regional traditions."

To save time and money and lose pounds, you should cook for yourself as much as possible, preferably most of the time.

When you factor in the extra pounds you'll likely put on by buying convenience foods, the last-minute shopping time, driving time, gas costs, and the financial and physical costs of unnecessary impulse items you also pick up, cooking at home totally beats convenience foods.

Cooking for yourself is faster, simpler, easier, and cheaper and helps you lose weight more quickly than relying on convenience foods, as long as you plan ahead and use some of my "secret" quick prep ideas, borrowed from all the restaurant kitchens I've worked in most of my life. For example:

When you cook at home, you have total control over the ingredients, and this is where I use my tricks of the trade to reinvent your favorite comfort foods—with fewer calories and less fat, sodium, and cholesterol. Healthful doesn't mean tasteless, either! I emphasize aromatics like garlic and onion, for example, Greek yogurt instead of sour cream, low-calorie seasonings, chicken stock that stands in for high-calorie oil, stevia in place of sugar, and "secret" cooking methods like flash-frying that let you have fried chicken (I'm not kidding!) but without all that nasty fat.

Rather than add carb-rich noodles to recipes, I like to use the newest low-carb food on the block: shirataki noodles. In case you're not familiar with these noodles, they're made from konnyaku, a dough of Asian yam (konjac) flour and water. Shirataki noodles are a superb pasta substitute; each serving has twenty calories or fewer, plus two grams of fiber. They're low on the glycemic index, too, so they won't send your blood sugar through the roof. Not only that, but they also have zero gluten—great news for those of you who can't tolerate that potential allergen.

THE BASICS OF QUICK, HEALTHY COOKING

What comes first, the recipe or the ingredients? This of course depends on your circumstances. It's always very helpful to walk into a store with a well-conceived list based on a recipe, but sometimes life does not allow that, now, does it?

If you want to make a healthier version of a dish you know and love, break it down into its essential parts and see where you can swap out unhealthy ingredients and swap in healthier ones that taste the same or will work the same physically or chemically to keep the final product the same. If you're running freestyle and conceiving a dish while shopping for the healthiest ingredients you can find, you should consider the following: The most important thing a dish should do is leave you with a feeling of fullness and satisfaction, so consider things that make you feel full without empty calories, like whole grains and fruits and veggies.

The fun part for me is creating flavor! Once you've selected your main ingredients, look at ways to create good flavor contrasts according to your mood. I like the following go-to items to boost flavors:

1. *Low-fat, low-sodium chicken stock in a box*

2. *Frozen vegetables and fruits*

3. *Canned foods like tomatoes, beets, beans, garbanzos, and lentils*

4. *Rotisserie chicken*

5. *Lemons and limes*

6. *Fresh herbs*

7. *Aromatics like garlic, ginger, and cocoa powder*

8. *Condiments like Dijon mustard, low-sugar ketchup, agave nectar, coconut nectar, and apple butter*

9. *Vinegars: red wine vinegar, white wine vinegar, balsamic vinegar, rice wine vinegar, and cider vinegar*

10. *Dried spices and herbs: nutmeg, allspice, cumin, chili powder, curry powder, black peppercorns, white peppercorns, dried thyme, dried oregano, dried rosemary, red chili flakes, paprika, Old Bay seasoning, sea salt*

To create sweetness, try raw fruit and vegetable juices, monk fruit (luo han guo), stevia, inulin natural sweetener products, raw agave, raw coconut nectar, raw coconut sugar, or fat-free milk powder. For something sour, add unsweetened vinegars, lemon juice, grapefruit juice, lime juice, green apples, pineapple, tamarind, or yogurt. And for bitterness, use unsweetened cocoa powder, instant espresso powder, mustard powder, chili powder, raw garlic, horseradish, wasabi powder, mustard, fresh chilis, tea leaves, roasted seaweed, toasted nuts, hot sauce, or spicy curry pastes.

If you want to add a salty taste, look for things that carry other natural flavor enhancers, like yeast extract or umami carriers. Your salt additions should give your dish a rounder, fully-flavored feel, helping your food hit all the flavor perceptors on your palate. Try low-sodium soy, Vegemite, Marmite, capers, anchovies, hard aged cheese, dry aged lean hams or beef, or miso. To add aroma, use herbs, spices, anything roasted or toasted, seeds, aromatic vegetables, smoked items, and extracts such as vanilla, almond, and citrus.

Conveniences of Life

There are great new shortcut products coming out all the time, like prepackaged sugar-free and low-sodium dips and salsas, and my favorite: the prepackaged fresh vegetable packs that have already peeled and cut vegetables, which make soups, stews, and stir-fries much easier and faster endeavors. I love using retail outlets for quick things, like steamed brown rice, fresh juices from juice bars, roasted chickens (which I peel the skin off of), and steamed shrimp.

MY FAVORITE HEALTHY COOKING TECHNIQUES TO PUNCH UP THE FLAVOR

- **Steaming:** A good way to cook vegetables and thinly sliced proteins. Good retention of nutrients. Use a steam basket or fold up aluminum foil into a rack to fit in the bottom of any pot.

- **Steam pockets:** Spread out aluminum foil and place ingredients in the center, fold up the sides, add a little liquid (stock, water, etc.), and fold the sides shut. Place the packet in a dry, hot sauté pan and let the steam inside puff the pocket out, then flip the pocket and steam the other side. Turn off the heat and cut the pocket open with scissors, being careful of the steam that will billow out of the cut. This works well with already-cooked produce that needs to reheat in a sauce, or small-cut seafood, vegetables, and tofu, or cooked noodle dishes.

- **Sautéing:** Use olive oil cooking spray (such as Pam) on a nonstick pan. If you don't have a nonstick sauté pan, place a thin coat of olive oil in a pan and heat over medium-high heat, then swab out the oil with a towel and proceed. *Caution:* When using cooking spray, it's very important to spray the pan first, then place over the heat—otherwise, you run the risk of a flame burst.

- **Broiling:** A very good option for cooking with little fat, broiling is pretty clean as well. Line a cookie sheet with aluminum foil and place a rack over the top, then set whatever you're going to broil on the rack. You can lightly spray the ingredients with cooking spray before broiling to enhance caramelization and even cooking. Use broiling for cutlets of any kind and thinner vegetables like asparagus or long stick cuts of vegetables like sweet potato fries or root vegetables.

- **Microwave:** I love the microwave, love it. Just be sure not to use plastic containers (I use Pyrex microwave-safe glass vessels), and if you're using plastic wrap, make sure it's labeled microwave safe—and to be extra safe, be sure it doesn't come in contact with the food. You can avoid plastic altogether by covering a Pyrex bowl with a microwave-safe plate.

- **Faux-frying:** Use whole-wheat flour, whipped egg whites, and whole-wheat panko bread crumbs for breading. Place food on a rack in a very hot oven.

- **Flash-frying:** The trick to flash-frying is to cook or poach the food before it goes in the fryer. For chicken, poach in broth, then when it's almost fully cooked, coat with buttermilk and whole-wheat flour before frying in grape-seed oil. It won't take long before you get a nice crusty coating.

- **Grilling:** No oil required. Just fire up the grill, or an indoor grill pan when it's too cold or rainy outside.

- **High-heat stovetop cooking:** In the old days, I'd heat my pan, then add oil, butter, or bacon fat before adding the ingredients. Now I simply heat the pan until very hot, remove the pan from the heat, spray with nonstick spray before adding ingredients, and then return the pan to the heat.

GIVE YOUR SALT SHAKER A REST

The problem: Most Americans consume way too much sodium, and way too little potassium, a combo that increases the risk of high blood pressure, heart disease, and death. Americans, on average, consume some 3,400 milligrams of sodium on a daily basis, but experts call for a maximum of 2,300 milligrams a day (only about a teaspoon of salt), and 1,500 milligrams a day (two-thirds of a teaspoon) for people who have high blood pressure or are at high risk of getting it, which means 70 percent of American adults—including people over forty, African Americans, and people with somewhat elevated blood pressure, or prehypertension.

You can easily blow through these maximum numbers for a whole day by having just a single restaurant meal—one restaurant chain's New England

Lobster and Clam Bake was recently reported as having over 6,000 milligrams of sodium! Huge quantities of sodium are often added to foods during processing. In fact, 75 percent of Americans' sodium intake comes from processed foods. The Salty Top 10 food sources of sodium in the US diet, based on consumption frequency and the combination of sodium content, are these items, most of which are processed in some form and have vast amounts of sodium dumped into them during processing:

1. *Meat pizza*

2. *White bread*

3. *Processed cheese*

4. *Hot dogs*

5. *Spaghetti with sauce*

6. *Ham*

7. *Ketchup*

8. *Cooked rice*

9. *White rolls*

10. *Flour tortillas*

The solution: Use salt sparingly when cooking at home. With most dishes, you really need only a little pinch of salt, or none at all. Maybe it's the Italian chef in me, but my dishes taste so good I rarely feel the urge to sprinkle anything on them at the table. But if you're one of those people who just has to enjoy the ritual shaking of a powdery substance over your plate, there a number of salt-free substitutes and herb and spice mixes you can try. Trust me. I predict they'll taste better than the salt, which you'll hardly miss after a few days.

In the grocery store, pay attention to sodium content listed on packages. Keep in mind that your total sodium consumption should be 1,500 to 2,300 milligrams per day. **And, when eating out, check the sodium stats on the menus.** If they're not available, ask the server why not, and ask for low-sodium options.

You can also dial down the sodium and crank up the potassium by adding more fresh produce to your diet. Potassium is high and sodium is low in many vegetables and fruits, which is the combo you want. Especially good sources of potassium are leafy green veggies like spinach, collards, and kale; orange veggies such as sweet potatoes and yams and winter squash, and citrus fruits like grapefruits and oranges. **Watch what happens when you switch out the processed foods:**

Food*	You Want Less Sodium, milligrams	You Want More Potassium, milligrams
White beans, cooked, 1 cup	11	1,004
Spinach, cooked, 1 cup	126	839
Sweet potato, cooked, 1/2 cup	36	475
Broccoli, cooked, 1 cup	64	457
Cantaloupe, cubes, 1 cup	26	427
Salmon, cooked, 3 ounces	49	369
Cherry tomatoes, 1 cup	7	353
Kale, cooked, 1 cup	30	296
Blackberries, 1 cup	1	233
Orange, 1 medium	1	232
Collard greens, cooked, 1 cup	30	220
Grapefruit, red, 1/2	0	166
Bacon, cooked, 2 slices	384	93
American cheese, 1-ounce slice	452	79
Hot dog, 1	513	70
Chicken vegetable soup, canned, 1 cup	972	159
Beef pot pie, frozen, 1 pie	978	308
Pepperoni pizza, 2 slices	1,365	372

* Note: Values on fresh foods assume no added salt in cooking or at the table.

Sources for sodium section: Harvard School of Public Health, USDA National Nutrient Database

FOR AN EXTRA WEIGHT LOSS EDGE

The big news in weight loss foods and appetite suppressants isn't pills, but foods: the low-calorie-density foods can help you lose weight and keep it off. And unfortunately, nobody has discovered an effective, safe over-the-counter weight loss pill or herbal supplement. No supplement has been proven to "burn fat" or "speed up your metabolism," at least not yet.

As the authors of a research review published in the April 2012 issue of the *International Journal of Sports Nutrition and Exercise Metabolism* pointed out, "There is no strong research evidence indicating that a specific supplement will produce significant weight loss (>2 kg), especially in the long term. Some foods or supplements such as green tea, fiber, and calcium supplements or dairy products may complement a healthy lifestyle to produce small weight losses or prevent weight gain over time. Weight loss supplements containing metabolic stimulants (e.g., caffeine, ephedra, synephrine) are most likely to produce adverse side effects and should be avoided."

But research indicates that there are some things that may give you a small advantage in the weight loss battle. The research is preliminary, and sometimes conflicting, but there are four promising foods and supplements that might give you a small edge, and I think we need every edge we can get!

- **A multivitamin, multimineral supplement:** The best way to get your nutrients is through healthy food. But a lot of us aren't eating as healthy as we should. Multis provide nutritional insurance, not as a weight loss aid but to complement your diet to ensure that your basic nutritional needs are met. I think it's a good idea to take an all-purpose multivitamin/mineral supplement. It's what I do every day.

- **Chili peppers:** They contain a group of chemicals called capsaicinoids that may, when consumed over time, increase calorie burn and reduce appetite. According to a major research review published in the October 2012 issue of the scientific journal *Appetite*, "capsaicinoids are not a magic bullet for weight loss; the evidence is that they could play a beneficial role, as part of a weight management program." My advice is to sprinkle chili peppers on your food whenever you're in the mood, not only because of the potential weight loss edge, but because they punch up lots of dishes and make food taste great.

- **Green tea:** There is some evidence that consumption of green tea and other teas like oolong and white tea might provide a small edge in your weight loss effort, perhaps from fat-metabolism-enhancing properties in caffeine or other components in the tea, like cate-chins. Personally, I like green tea because of its clean, crisp taste, and if it's giving me a calorie-burning boost, hey, I'll take it!

- **White kidney bean extract:** Shows promise as a carb blocker in slowing and blocking the absorption of refined carbohydrates in the gastrointestinal tract and decreasing appetite. "Animal and human studies clearly show that this agent works," according to an article by Professor Harry Preuss of the Department of Medi-cine and Pathology at Georgetown University in the *Journal of the American College of Nutrition* (June 2009). If you're interested, consult with your doctor.

LOVE WHAT YOU EAT

I know a lot of people who think of a weight loss diet as being based on self-torture, denial, anxiety, and giving up lots of their favorite foods. But I strongly believe that the words *give up* should be at the top of your "don't do" list. Don't give up things. Don't ever use the sentence "I have to give up this food." There are ways to enjoy all your favorite things. They may just have to be reconfigured. I don't think you can give up your favorite foods and be successful on a diet. It's never going to happen. I don't believe you can be successful in maintaining a healthy diet by denying yourself the things you love over the long term. If you grew up loving red meat and potatoes and ketchup your whole life and you suddenly say, "I can never eat them again for the rest of my life," I don't think that's going to work.

My whole approach is based on reconfiguring your favorite foods so you can enjoy them. I do it for you in this book. Rather than give up the foods you've loved your whole life, you have to shift away from the versions of them that aren't good for you and start to create new versions of them. Any dish can be transformed from an unhealthy version to a healthy version—and in most cases you won't taste what you're missing. And you can absolutely do this at home. Just in Twitter conversations, I've heard thousands of people telling me "Oh, I make a healthy this, a healthy that."

I don't think you necessarily need to give up alcohol forever, if you don't have a problem with drinking. I think it's a really good idea to reduce the amount you drink, because the calorie impact can be significant over time, but I think for most people a glass of wine or beer here and there is part of life, and there's a way to keep it in your life without derailing your weight.

Having read my previous books about healthy weight loss, a lot of people are telling me it's a lot easier than they expected, especially with the help of my recipes. They're always surprised at how good the recipes are. They're exhilarated by the immediate results in how they look and feel, and how rapid the weight loss can be.

I'm hearing a lot about the joy of cooking at home, about the joy of getting back into the kitchen, about people reconnecting with their family, the husbands, wives, children, how people are enjoying entertaining. How even people who live alone are enjoying cooking for themselves, how they feel empowered, in control.

As a chef, I look at healthy dieting as the manipulation of three things: mouth-feel, belly-feel, and body-feel. Mouth-feel is flavor, so that eating is a joyful experience. Belly-feel is satisfaction, so that you're full and happy, and not prompted to gorge on too much food. And body-feel is how much energy your body feels all day long.

What I do with my food, because of the combination of my culinary skills and my interest in health and wellness, is to create the most satisfaction per calorie of food, versus the average chef or diet expert. So in terms of feeling full, that's not an issue. You're not going to feel hungry on any of the dishes I produce because there is so much satisfaction for the number of calories. In terms of feeling full, the satisfaction level is definitely there. Highly flavorful foods that taste exciting are much more fulfilling.

On every level, you're going to feel full, feel the excitement that you get from eating great food. Food has to be built for flavor. That's something I did with my first cookbook. It was called **Flavor**. I'm all about creating that intense relationship with sour, salty, sweet, and bitter. There's excitement, a buildup, and resolution; my food is like good music. You're not going to feel like you're missing out on anything. It's not going to feel like punishment! It's something you can do for a long time and it's not going to feel any different than what you've been doing.

The correct definition of a diet is a natural, enjoyable, healthy eating pattern you follow for the rest of your life. Along with regular physical activity, it will help keep you at a healthy weight. A diet is a pattern to be enjoyed, not a straitjacket to suffer in.

Have you ever EWI—Eaten While Impaired? Eating While Impaired means eating when you're too hungry, like when you've skipped meals or you're on too restrictive a diet, with too many hard-to-follow rules. I'll tell you what happens to me when I sometimes EWI.

I binge. I pork out. I stuff my face with too much food.

It seems the longer I go without regular, satisfying full meals, at least one meal or healthy snack every three hours or so, the more I overeat. This simple physical dynamic, EWI, is why I think most diets are doomed to fail, by definition. They're just too darn hard to follow.

Not long ago, the World Health Organization asked a superstar panel of the world's greatest scientific, medical, and research experts on the subjects of diet and nutrition a simple question: What strategies work for weight loss?

Their answer: What **won't work** is eating patterns based on "rigid restraint and periodic disinhibition." In other words, strict rules usually don't work, because we'll break them sooner or later, guaranteed. What will work, they concluded, is "flexible restraint." A healthy, sustainable diet is a **pattern** of healthy eating, a rhythm that you maintain naturally through the course of the days, weeks, and months.

If you eat a less than perfectly healthy meal now and then, it's OK! Forgive yourself! What matters most isn't the unhealthy meal you scarf down one time as you're trying to lose weight; what matters most is the **overall pattern** of what you eat over time.

You want a diet plan that delivers results quickly enough for you to stay motivated and inspired, but a plan that is based on good science and healthy nutrition, not on wacky theories or self-appointed medical gurus or quacks you read about on the Internet. You need a diet based on indulgence, not on torturing yourself, a diet based on flavor, satisfaction, and a full, happy belly.

The Skinny on Weight Loss Success

When I started Rocco's diet I was 180 pounds, and today I am 133.8. I never thought I could be 133. And now I realize I could even be probably 125. The experience was fabulous!

Rocco's recipes are amazing, tasty and incredibly savory. He's worked out all the calorie numbers. I never felt deprived. I was never hungry, not once. My only complaint is my closet is filled with all these baggy clothes. I still can't believe I've lost all this weight.

A couple of my girlfriends and I went shopping, since everything I put on at home was hanging off me. I was trying on size 14s because that used to be my size. The saleslady kept bringing me smaller and smaller sizes. I was putting on 12s, 10s, 8s, even size 6 was too big. I finally wound up with size 4!

For me, it was Rocco to the rescue! He really has the key to success with this diet! He introduces you to a journey of mindful eating. He's done all the hard work for you. All you need to do is just believe and do it.

—Rochelle

CHAPTER 10

On Your Way

CONGRATULATIONS on your new lifestyle!

I'm so proud of you!

I really encourage you to take the principles of this book to heart, and to stick with them.

Believe me, I know what it's like to be overweight and feel really bad about it, but today I know the spectacular feeling of being lean and healthy. Once you get that feeling, I bet you'll never want to give it up.

Don't ever forget the wonderful health benefits that come to you when you live and eat this way.

You'll live longer, more happily, and more actively. You'll be around longer for your kids and your significant other—to laugh with them, savor delicious food with them, and chase them around more. And chances are you'll stay out of the hospital more and you won't have to take bucketfuls of medicine and pills every day—all because you decided to eat right and get physically active.

What inspired you to do this in the first place was the promise of a diet that wasn't a diet, but a lifestyle you could fall in love with over the long term.

It's a beautiful dream, and it can absolutely come true for you!

Remember: The diet that will work best for you is the healthy eating pattern that you can enjoy over the long term. And that's exactly what I've given you.

Staying lean and healthy is a lifelong process of staying aware, and of periodic monitoring of yourself—your weight and other health stats.

Your weight may go up and down a bit, especially around holiday seasons, and you might slide down the slippery slope of losing your inhibitions now and then and find yourself putting on weight. It can creep on slowly and quietly and then suddenly, BANG! You've put on too much!

It's OK! Forgive yourself! I've been there myself and I know how bad it can feel. You can sit around and feel miserable, and lament, "Why did I let this happen to me? I can't get out of this bind!"

Sure you can.

Just go back to the basic principles we've explored in this book, and you'll get back on track.

And remember why you decided to eat and live healthy—so you'll be alive, happy, and healthy for your family, your children, your friends, and all the people who count on you!

I'd love to know how you're making out with your journey to health and weight control. Why don't you tell the world how you're doing and what you've learned, on my Facebook page—facebook.com/RoccoDiSpirito.

AFTERWORD

The Lesson of the Apple

·

ONE OF THE best secrets for losing weight is to stick to a plant-based diet of whole foods.

And whenever you can, I suggest you choose fresh, locally grown food, and I suggest you support your local farmers and farmers' markets. As a chef, I've supported farmers' markets and local, sustainable sources of food for many years. As an advocate, I've testified for food banks and lobbied for food security before Congress. As a member of the community, I've helped run food pantries to lend a hand to families in trouble. And today I have a food truck on the streets of New York that serves fresh, low-calorie food and visits public schools to educate children on healthy eating, sustainability, and food security.

When politicians talk, do you get as confused as I do? Tax policy, health care, the economy—do you walk away even more confused because of the political rhetoric—and the clash of statistics? Well, on the subject of food in America there is no debate—we have become trapped in what I call a circle of madness. Consider these horrifying facts:

- Obesity now affects 17 percent of all children and adolescents in the United States—triple the rate from just one generation ago.

- More than one-third of American adults are obese.

- Obesity-related conditions are sharply rising and include heart disease, stroke, type 2 diabetes, and certain types of cancer, some of the leading causes of preventable death.

- Medical costs associated with obesity were recently estimated at almost $147 billion.

- At the same time, millions of American families and children, or almost 15 percent of our households, experienced food insecurity during 2011, and our food pantries are overwhelmed.

Something is terribly wrong. It really is a circle of madness. Through the buying decisions we make every single day, we are empowering gigantic companies to produce heavily processed, genetically modified foods from such tiny pieces of land that such production was never considered humanly possible. And we have more people hungry today that we've ever had in the history of our country. None of the choices we're making as a nation are producing results we're happy with. The irony is that we're supposed to be the richest country in the world, and we produce the most food—but we can't feed our own people!

As the saying goes, everything is connected. Let's take energy independence, for example. Can you imagine how much less fuel our cars and planes would use if Americans weren't the most obese people in the world? There is a direct relationship between your weight and the gas consumption of your car! How about genetically modified foods? Industrial farming and the advances in agritechnology have done nothing to help us end hunger or help increase food security in any way, and they've done nothing to make us healthier.

I am convinced that the high incidence of gluten intolerance today is specifically the result of hybridized wheat, GMO wheat that's producing near-toxic levels of gluten, and for many people may be triggering digestive problems, autism, and weight gain. It's all connected.

Local, sustainable food is key to a healthy diet. How do you think our fruits and vegetables could possibly survive a five-thousand-mile trip? Drugs! They're being shot up and bathed in hormones, chemicals, colorants, and Lord knows what else. It's science fiction; it's like a horror movie. Don't kid yourself about the food you eat. When food has five thousand miles on it, it no longer is what it was when it started. It might be less expensive, or it might be available off season, but it's just not going to provide the nutrition it would have originally.

It's time we put a stop to all this. It's time we demand that food and restaurant companies stop the excuses and figure out how to deliver the healthiest, most delicious food and meals to us. That means they must cut way down on the bad fats, the bad carbs, the added sugars, the excessive sodium, and the elephant-sized portions—and crank up the good carbs, the whole grains, the good fats, the fresh produce, the healthy herbs and spices, and most of all, the taste. We must vote with our pocketbooks and reward those companies that do it right. Don't let them BS you about how hard it is to make healthy food taste great—it does take extra work and it is somewhat harder to figure out, but I do it every day in my book recipes and my food truck.

When you're out there shopping for food, find out where it was grown. Buy local whenever you can. If you're a New Yorker and it was grown in Pennsylvania or Vermont or upstate New York, it's local to you. It wasn't grown in Belgium or China or Mexico. It hasn't traveled five thousand miles to get to you—and it's still food!

If we look to the hippies of the 1960s, if we look to the Italians of today, if we look to a lot of Third World countries where people eat local, fresh, sustainable food and home-cooked meals—all the lessons we need to learn are right there in front of us. It's all about eating a largely plant-based diet of whole foods that are grown locally, prepared at home, and harvested, sold, prepared, and eaten within a few hundred miles.

What else do we need to know? It has to start at home. Children model your behavior more than they listen to words. Switch off the TV, turn off the video games and smartphone, go outside and play with them on the grass, and come home and cook together. You can make change happen instantaneously with every decision you make for your family in a grocery store—stick to the fresh food sections, shop the perimeter of the store, stay away from the packaged and processed food aisles. Do not buy processed foods. If you have to buy something that has to be slipped into a foil-cardboard sheath, then microwaved, then turned upside down after two minutes—you're probably not making a very good choice for your family!

It's always amazing to me how many parents will strictly monitor their children's video game and TV habits, and will interview potential playdate partners, yet they will teach their children unhealthy food habits, leading to our being the most obese developed nation in the world, where early-onset diabetes among children is at epidemic proportions.

It all starts at home. Go and buy some fresh local food, cook it for your family, and enjoy the process—it's wonderful! I do it every single day of my life, and I'm as busy as anybody. If you think you're powerless and you can't make change happen—guess what? We've totally got the power.

A while ago, I gave up apples. They bored me. They tasted bland. They didn't taste like apples anymore. They tasted unripe and rotten—because of the way they were grown and shipped. I'd become jaded. I stopped eating apples, one of the greatest things you can do for your health. An apple a day really does keep the doctor away, and I recommend three a day!

The other day I bought an apple at the farmers' market. It had been grown about a hundred miles from New York City. It was cheap, and it was one of the most delicious apples I've ever tasted! I was so happy to find that the locally grown option tasted so good. I went back and bought a bunch more, everyone in my house started eating them, and now I can't keep count of how many we're putting away. They're under a hundred calories each—they're a terrific snack! That's just one example of how we consumers have all the power.

These are problems that are so easily solved. You don't need to vote on it. You don't need to start a group. You don't need to rally people and get petitions signed. All you have to do is go to the grocery store and make a choice that tells the buyers what you want. And they'll respond.

Why are there farmers' markets now in urban areas where there weren't any twenty years ago? Why is there a Whole Foods Market? Why does Whole Foods Market tell you where they grow their food? Because it's important to know and we've empowered them with our buying decisions.

Understand that you can effect change instantaneously, tomorrow morning, with the choices you make. The breakfast you eat, where you go for lunch, where you shop, and what you buy can change the world. That's how you make change happen. It's so easy. We have the power.

You can't change foreign policy when you wake up tomorrow morning. You can't change economic policy when you wake up tomorrow morning. But we can change this! We should be thrilled! We're always looking for places in our lives where we can help change the world for the better. Well, this is the place, and now is the time to put these principles into action. We can lose weight, live longer and healthier lives, and make the world a better place to live in.

We can make it happen.

I wish you lots of love, laughter, a very happy belly, and great success with your weight loss journey. Now let's go out there and lose weight, keep it off, and change the world—one locally grown apple at a time!

RESOURCES

My Top Websites for Weight Control, Health, and Nutrition Information

www.calorieking.com

Excellent source for calorie counts for a wide variety of foods.

www.myfitnesspal.com

Estimated calorie burns for many different physical activities.

www.mayoclinic.com

Great health information from the Mayo Clinic, a trusted source.

www.webmd.com

Lots more great health information from another trusted authority.

www.hsph.harvard.edu/nutritionsource/

The Harvard School of Public Health, good info on a wide variety of nutrition and weight control topics.

www.pubmed.com

A superb government website that indexes a huge number of research papers on health, fitness, nutrition, and weight loss published in peer-reviewed medical and scientific journals. An excellent filter to bypass the oceans of bad information on the Internet and get to the good stuff.

www.choosemyplate.gov/SuperTracker/

Exactly how many calories you should consume to maintain or lose weight can be a complex subject that can depend on your sex, height, weight, body type, and activity level. This is a good, free US government website for calculating your personalized daily calorie target that takes these variables into account, with a program called the SuperTracker. Let's say you're a thirty-five-year-old American woman who is around the average height and weight, 5 feet 4 inches and 163 pounds; is not breastfeeding or pregnant; and does an average of less than thirty minutes per day of moderate-intensity physical activity. The bad news: According to the BMI chart, you're overweight, because you have a 28 BMI. The good news: You've got an estimated "magic number" to shoot for. According to the SuperTracker, on average, to move down to a healthy weight, you should eat **1,800 calories a day**. If you wanted to get to a healthy weight faster, you would eat even fewer calories a day and add in physical activity, or do some combination of both.

If you're a man of thirty-five who is around the average height and weight, 5 feet 9 inches and 190 pounds, and does an average of less than thirty minutes per day of moderate-intensity physical activity, the bad news is that according to the BMI chart, you're overweight because you also have a 28 BMI. The good news: According to the SuperTracker, on average, to move down to a healthy weight, you should eat **2,400 calories a day**. If you wanted to get to a healthy weight faster, you would eat even fewer calories a day and add in physical activity, or do some combination of both.

Additional notes on weight loss: Kevin D. Hall, PhD, of the National Institutes of Health argued in a 2008 paper in the *International Journal of Obesity* ("What Is the Required Energy [calorie] Deficit per Unit Weight Loss?") that while the "3500 calorie deficit = 1 pound of weight loss" formula could be accurate for some people, "a larger cumulative energy deficit [calorie deficit] is required per unit weight loss for people with greater initial body fat," which may explain "why men can lose more weight than women for a given energy deficit [calorie deficit] since women typically have more body fat than men of similar body weight." In a 2011 paper in *The Lancet* ("Quantifying the Effect of Energy Imbalance on Body Weight Change"), Hall and his colleagues presented an online Body Weight Simulator tool you may want to check out with your doctor. The simulator estimates body weight changes over time with different levels of calories and physical activity. Find the simulator at bwsimulator.niddk.nih.gov/.

Also, the authors of a 2008 article in the journal *Obesity*, "Successful Weight Loss Maintenance in Relation to Method of Weight Loss," pointed out that the definition of a very-low-calorie diet is arbitrary and can vary depending on the person: "A 700 kcal/d [calories per day] diet, for example, would induce a relatively modest energy [calorie] deficit in a short, sedentary woman with a resting energy [calorie] expenditure (REE) of 1100 kcal/d.

In contrast, a 1200 kcal/d diet would induce a substantial energy [calorie] deficit in a tall man with an REE of 2500 kcal/d. The man would seem to have a greater risk of adverse metabolic effects…even though technically he was prescribed an LCD and the woman a VLCD. Thus, an alternative definition of a VLCD is a diet that provides <50% of an individual's predicted REE."

Resources for Recipe "Before" Nutritional Information

BREAKFAST RECIPES

Protein-Packed Breakfast Sandwich

http://caloriecount.about.com/calories-mcdonalds-sausage-egg-cheese -mcgriddles-i84420

All-Day Egg-White Omelet with Pico de Gallo

www.walmart.com/ip/Jimmy-Dean-Ham-Cheese-Omelets-8.6-oz/ 12444401#Nutrition+Facts

Greek Yogurt with Crunchy Blueberry Topping

www.food.com/recipe/a-breakfast-yogurt-parfait-granola-130766

Instant Oatmeal with Psychedelic Fruit Crispies

http://caloriecount.about.com/calories-mcdonalds-fruit-maple-oatmeal -i194709

Apple Cinnamon Crunch Cereal

http://tracker.dailyburn.com/nutrition/cinnamon_toast_crunch_with _whole_milk_calories

Grapefruit with Zero-Calorie Spiced "Sugar"

http://recipes.sparkpeople.com/recipe-calories.asp?recipe=2463217

BEVERAGE RECIPES

Banana Cream Smoothie

www.calorieking.com/foods/calories-in-beverages-smoothies-banana _f-ZmlkPTE3NDIoMg.html

The Green Monkey
www.incrediblesmoothies.com/recipes/banana-smoothie-recipes-and
-nutrition/

Southern-Style Sweet Tea
www.myfitnesspal.com/food/calories/mcdonalds-sweet-tea-large-44174117

Mexican Hot Chocolate
http://caloriecount.about.com/calories-swiss-miss-hot-chocolate-mix-i114499

Green Tea with Lemon and Basil
www.myfitnesspal.com/food/calories/mcdonalds-sweet-tea-large-44174117

Ginger Boost Peach Smoothie
www.chick-fil-a.com/Food/Menu-Detail/Peach-Milkshake#?details=
nutrition

High-Protein Chocolate Breakfast Smoothie
http://recipes.sparkpeople.com/recipe-detail.asp?recipe=1385412

Virgin Mary
http://caloriecount.about.com/calories-red-lobster-bloody-mary-i168033

Almond Milk Smoothie
www.myfitnesspal.com/food/calories/cyndis-homemade-almond-milk
-blueberry-almond-butter-protein-shake-25014719

APPETIZER, SIDE, AND SNACK RECIPES

Fresh Wasabi Peas
www.caloriegallery.com/foods/calories-in-mishima-wasabi-green-peas.htm

Sweet Potato Chips
www.calorieking.com/foods/calories-in-potato-chips-krinkle-cut-salt
-fresh-ground-pepper_f-ZmlkPTEwMjU3NA.html

Crispy Hot and Sweet Garbanzos
www.food.com/recipe/fried-garbanzo-beans-335352

Super Popcorn-Kale Crumble
www.myfitnesspal.com/food/calories/movie-theater-popcorn-medium
-bag-with-butter-15669325#

Apples and Cheddar Cheese

www.food.com/recipe/baked-brie-in-puff-pastry-with-apricot-or-raspberry
-preserves-48907

SOUP AND SALAD RECIPES

Mushroom Miso Noodle Soup

www.myfitnesspal.com/food/calories/woerz-homemade-chicken-noodle
-soup-egg-noodles-chicken-carrots-mushrooms-celary-5485844

Mediterranean Tuna Salad

http://caloriecount.about.com/calories-tuna-salad-i15128

Turkey and Lentil Soup

www.livestrong.com/thedailyplate/nutrition-calories/food/soup-bible
-homemade/lentil-and-bacon-soup/

Tomato and Shrimp Kimchi Salad

www.myfitnesspal.com/food/calories/chopt-roasted-shrimp-salad
-with-spinach-tomato-cucumber-beets-and-white-balsamic-vinaigrette
-41992153

Tomato and Vegetable Soup

www.food.com/recipe/tomato-noodle-soup-198043

Old-Fashioned Chicken Noodle Soup

www.calorieking.com/foods/calories-in-soups-chilis-chunky-chicken
-noodle-bowl_f-ZmlkPTE2NTgwNA.html

Calamari and Watermelon Salad

http://tracker.dailyburn.com/nutrition/japanese_salad_at_restaurant
_fried_calamari_salad_calories

Salmon and Cucumber Salad with Creamy Dill Dressing

www.calorieking.com/foods/calories-in-salads-grilled-salmon-caesar
-with-spicy-dressing_f-ZmlkPTE4NzUoMg.html

Crunchy Kale, Apple, and Pomegranate Salad

www.myfitnesspal.com/food/calories/true-foods-restaurant-raw-tuscan
-kale-salad-47352627

Grilled Shrimp Gazpacho

www.myfitnesspal.com/food/calories/sodexo-workplace-gazpacho
-anduluz-8-oz-39396000

Manhattan Clam Chowder

www.bhg.com/recipe/soups/manhattan-clam-chowder/

Black Bean and Chicken Mole

www.myfitnesspal.com/food/calories/safeway-cafe-baked-chicken-flautas
-with-chile-peanut-mole-mango-black-bean-salsa-rice-mexican-crema
-45167893

Southwestern Rice and Bean Salad with Cheddar Cheese

www.fatsecret.com/calories-nutrition/taco-bell/cheesy-bean-and-rice-burrito

MAIN COURSE RECIPES

Rotisserie Chicken and Teriyaki Asian Noodles

http://www.wolfgangpuck.com/content/files/foodmenu_RWC%20Nutrition%
20Spreadsheet%2010-3-11.pdf

Thai Noodles with Turkey

www.bettycrocker.com/recipes/thai-peanut-chicken-and-noodles/
edaacafe-4700-4c9f-860b-c09afeb881d5

Turkey Alfredo

www.olivegarden.com/menu/nutrition/

Salisbury Steak with Mushroom Gravy

http://allrecipes.com/recipe/salisbury-steak/

Lemon Garlic Shrimp Pasta

www.food.com/recipe/lemon-garlic-shrimp-over-pasta-145738

Beef and Broccoli Stir-Fry

www.myfitnesspal.com/food/calories/panda-express-panda-bowl-fried
-rice-and-broccoli-beef-33465737

Roasted Turkey with Green Beans and Gravy

http://caloriecount.about.com/calories-ruby-tuesday-roasted-turkey
-gravy-i54963

Sweet Sesame Turkey with Bok Choy

http://tindrumcafe.com/nutritional_information.pdf

Vegetable Egg Rolls with Chia-Chili Sauce

http://calorielab.com/restaurants/original-roadhouse-grill/texas-egg
-rolls/364/41107

Pork Cutlet alla Pizzaiola

www.colavita.com/recipesArchive/recipe.cfm?id=2048

RD's Big Burger with All the Fixin's

www.bk.com/en/us/menu-nutrition/lunch-and-dinner-menu-202/flame
-broiled-burgers-220/whopper-sandwich-m1/index.html

Bacon-Wrapped Chicken with Sweet Rutabaga Mash

http://allrecipes.com/recipe/bacon-wrapped-chicken/

BBQ Chicken Cutlets

www.famousdaves.com/contact/nutrition-and-allergy-information

Chicken Cheesesteak with Jalapeños

www.calorieking.com/foods/calories-in-sandwiches-burgers-sub-8
-chipotle-cheesesteak-chicken-on-wheat-bread_f-ZmlkPTE4MzAzMA
.html

Chicken Enchiladas

www.kraftrecipes.com/recipes/chicken-sour-cream-enchiladas-51104
.aspx#

Crab Taco with Pico de Gallo and Cilantro

www.sparkpeople.com/calories-in.asp?food=don+pablos+fried+fish+tacos

Garlicky Shrimp and Spinach in a Foil Pouch

http://calorielab.com/restaurants/chin-chin/shrimp-with-black-beans/
4023/24605

Roasted Scrod with Vegetable Curry

www.food.com/recipe/pf-changs-coconut-curry-vegetables-400949

Salmon Teriyaki with Grapefruit and Fennel

www.myfitnesspal.com/food/calories/bento-nouveau-teriyaki-salmon
-rice-bowl-16891298

DESSERT RECIPES

High-Protein "Rice" Pudding with Papaya

www.fatsecret.com/calories-nutrition/generic/pudding-rice

Instant Vanilla Frozen Yogurt in a Blender

www.calorieking.com/foods/calories-in-ice-cream-original-vanilla
_f-ZmlkPTEwNDk5Mw.html

Instant Chocolate Soft-Serve in a Juicer

www.fatsecret.com/calories-nutrition/usda/rich-chocolate-ice-cream

Rocco's Quick-Fill Chocolate-Strawberry Bar

http://caloriecount.about.com/calories-clif-bar-chocolate-chip-i86848

Fresh Raspberries with Sugar-Free Vanilla Cream

http://www.calorieking.com/foods/calories-in-ice-creams-soft-serve
-parfait-made-with-m-ms_f-ZmlkPTE2MzIyMg.html

Fresh Strawberries with Sugar-Free Chocolate Sauce

http://www.sparkpeople.com/calories-in.asp?food=chocolate+dipped+stra
wberries

INDEX

ABOUT ROCCO DISPIRITO

ROCCO DISPIRITO is a chef and the author of nine previous award-winning books, including the #1 *New York Times* bestsellers **Now Eat This!** and **Now Eat This! Diet**.

Rocco's **Now Eat This!** series features healthy makeovers of America's favorite comfort foods, from fried chicken to apple pie, all with zero bad carbs, zero bad fats, zero sugar, and maximum flavor. Every dish weighs in at less than 350 calories. The series also includes the *New York Times* bestseller **Now Eat This! Italian.**

Rocco began his culinary studies at the Culinary Institute of America at the age of sixteen and by age twenty was working in the kitchens of legendary chefs around the globe. He was named *Food & Wine* magazine's Best New Chef and was the first chef to appear on *Gourmet* magazine's cover as "America's Most Exciting Young Chef." His three-star restaurant, Union Pacific, was a New York City culinary landmark for many years. In her famous *New York Times* review, restaurant critic Ruth Reichl said of her experience at Union Pacific, "I have yet to taste anything on Mr. DiSpirito's menu that is not wonderful. I was moaning as I ate."

Chef Rocco DiSpirito is on a mission to change people's perception of healthy food by making delicious low-fat, low-calorie dishes easily accessible. To that end, he launched the **Now Eat This! Truck,** which travels around New York City selling meals created from recipes featured in his successful series of cookbooks of the same name. Chef DiSpirito donates 100% of the proceeds to provide free lunches and nutrition education to New York City students. Once a week, during Free Lunch Fridays, Chef DiSpirito personally visits a different city school to educate the students on the benefits of eating healthy foods. As part of that program, he serves free lunches to the participating students, paid for by the generosity of other New Yorkers who buy their lunch from the **Now Eat This! Truck**.

His syndicated TV show **Now Eat This! with Rocco DiSpirito** began airing in 2012. His reality series, **Rocco's Dinner Party**, aired on Bravo. Rocco is a frequent guest on *Good Morning America*, *The Rachael Ray Show*, and *The Dr. Oz Show* and has appeared on *The View*, *Today*, *The Doctors*, *The Ellen DeGeneres Show*, and many other programs.